IMMUNOLOGY AND IMMUNE SYSTEM DISORDERS

# SJÖGREN'S SYNDROME

# SYMPTOMS, TREATMENT OPTIONS AND POTENTIAL HEALTH COMPLICATIONS

# IMMUNOLOGY AND IMMUNE SYSTEM DISORDERS

Additional books in this series can be found on Nova's website under the Series tab.

Additional e-books in this series can be found on Nova's website under the e-book tab.

IMMUNOLOGY AND IMMUNE SYSTEM DISORDERS

# SJÖGREN'S SYNDROME

# SYMPTOMS, TREATMENT OPTIONS AND POTENTIAL HEALTH COMPLICATIONS

EDUARDO M. HERNANDEZ
EDITOR

NOVA BIOMEDICAL

*New York*

For permission to use material from this book please contact us:
Telephone 631-231-7269; Fax 631-231-8175
Web Site: http://www.novapublishers.com



**Library of Congress Cataloging-in-Publication Data**

ISBN: 978-1-63117-859-7

*Published by Nova Science Publishers, Inc. † New York*

# Contents

# Preface

Sjögren's syndrome (SS) is a multi-system exocrinopathy. Its etiology remains unknown and it has an autoimmune pathogenesis. Although SS has been reported in young children and men, it is more frequent in middle-aged women. SS may occur alone, defined as primary SS, or in association with another autoimmune disease, defined as secondary SS. SS has a wide variety of glandular and extra-glandular manifestations affecting almost every organ. Despite its apparently inoffensive initial manifestations, SS can become a disabling and potentially life-threatening disease. This book discusses Sjögren's syndrome in detail, and provides further insight on topics that include the clinical manifestation and management of SS; the symptoms and diagnosis; health related quality of life in patients with SS; the involvement SS has in the central nervous system; and new aspects of mechanism of salivary glans dysfunctions in SS.

Chapter I – Objective: To describe the relationship between intake of omega-3 fatty acids (ω3) and symptom severity in patients with primary Sjogren's Syndrome.

Methods: This exploratory cross-sectional study recruited adult Sjogren's patients during routine office visits to a faculty rheumatology practice, when subjects provided data on their diet during the previous year, reported their current symptoms, and gave consent for investigators to review their medical records to ascertain prescribed therapy for Sjogren's syndrome. Patients completed a previously validated semi-quantitative food-frequency questionnaire, and they reported symptom severity (ocular sicca, oral sicca and overall Sjogren's-related symptoms) on three separate visual analog scales ranging from 0 to 100 (lowest to highest severity). A standard nutritional table indicating the ω3 content of common foods was applied to the food frequency data to estimate average daily ω3 consumption. Spearman's correlation coefficient was used to test the relationship between ω3 intake and symptom severity in patients receiving secretagogue therapy (e.g., cevimeline or pilocarpine), as well as in untreated patients. The Kruskal-Wallis test was used to compare symptom severity in 3 groups: pharmacologically treated patients, untreated patients reporting high intake of ω3 (≥500mg/d), and untreated patients reporting low intake of ω3 (<500mg/d).

Results: Among the 30 study subjects, the average daily intake of ω3 was 495±780mg/d (mean±SD). The average ocular, oral, and overall symptom severity scores were 56±29, 61±31, and 60±29, respectively. None of the correlations between ω3 intake and symptom severity were statistically significant ($p<0.05$) in either pharmacologically treated patients (n=12) or untreated patients (n=18). The mean ocular severity scores were 56, 53, and 57 in treated patients, untreated high-intake patients (n=6), and untreated low-intake patients (n=12), respectively. The corresponding oral severity scores were 56, 49, and 72, and the overall severity scores were 55, 49, and 70. While none of the differences in symptom severity across the 3 groups were statistically significant, the results do suggest possible beneficial effects of high ω3 intake for oral and overall symptoms that are roughly equivalent to the benefits of secretagogue therapy.

Conclusion: This exploratory investigation suggests the possibility that high intake of ω3 may have a beneficial effect on symptoms in patients with primary Sjogren's Syndrome who are not receiving secretagogue therapy. A larger study is needed to confirm or reject this hypotheses. A confirmatory result would make it worth considering ω3 supplementation as an alternative to pharmacologic therapy.

Chapter II – Primary Sjögren's syndrome (PSS) is a multi-system, immune-mediated, condition of unknown aetiology characterized by dryness of the eyes and mouth, pain and disabling fatigue. Other organs such as the skin, the nervous system, the lungs and the kidneys can also be affected. PSS is also associated with a markedly increased risk of lymphoma development. The health-related quality of life of patients with PSS is significantly impaired and the direct and indirect health economic cost associated with the condition is substantial.

The true prevalence of PSS is unknown but is estimated to be between 0.1-0.4% of the adult population with a strong female bias. The diagnosis is often delayed with PSS patients presenting to their doctors after suffering from the symptoms for many years. Improved links between rheumatologists, ophthalmologists, oral medicine specialists, dentists, opticians, and general practitioners can facilitate early diagnosis and reduce risk of long-term disability.

The American European Consensus Group (AECG) classification criteria 2002 are the current gold standard for the classification of PSS, although provisional American College of Rheumatology (ACR) criteria have recently been published. The development of consensus criteria by the ACR-European League Against Rheumatism (EULAR) working group to bring together the two criteria is in progress. Additionally, salivary gland ultrasound may also be an important component of the diagnostic criteria in the near future. Salivary gland sialometry, sialochemistry, tear osmolarity may be useful adjuncts, and the discovery of new diagnostic biomarkers is an area of active research.

Optimal assessment of patients with PSS, should encompass not only objective parameters such as abnormalities in blood tests and changes in tear and salivary flow, but also patient-reported outcome measures and impact on quality of life. Symptoms of PSS are often non-specific, therefore these symptoms must be actively explored. The recent development of EULAR outcome measurement tools for the assessment of systemic disease activity and patient-reported outcome has greatly facilitated standardised assessment of PSS in clinics and in research.

Management of PSS can be broadly classified into interventions targeting the glandular or systemic manifestations of the disease. Evidence-based strategies in PSS management remain elusive, instead, treatments are often based on empirical evidence or experience of the treating clinicians. The effective management of fatigue remains a major challenge. Recent advances in the understanding of PSS pathogenesis have led to the study of several biological therapies for the PSS with some encouraging data. Finally, optimal management of patients with PSS requires expertise from different disciplines such as ophthalmology, oral medicine and restorative dentistry.

Chapter III – Sjögren's syndrome (SS) is a multi-system exocrinopathy. Its etiology remains unknown and it has an autoimmune pathogenesis. Although SS has been reported in young children and men, it is more frequent in middle-aged women, with a sex ratio of 9:1. SS may occur alone, defined as primary SS, or in association with another autoimmune disease, defined as secondary SS. SS has a wide variety of glandular and extra-glandular manifestations affecting almost every organ. Despite its apparently inoffensive initial manifestations, SS can become a disabling and potentially life-threatening disease. Glandular manifestations vary according to the gland in question. The best predictor for SS is dry mouth (xerostomia), the most common SS symptom, followed by dry eyes. The low salivary flow increases susceptibility to bacterial and fungal diseases and often results in oral candidiasis. Dry eye (keratoconjunctivitissicca) is the most common ocular symptom. The main systemic manifestations are fatigue, dry airways, dry skin, dry vagina, dyspepsia, peripheral neuropathies, and autoimmune thyroiditis. Lymphoma, mostly of mucosa-associated lymphoid tissue type, is a characteristic but unusual feature that appears in approximately 5% of SS patients. The multiple manifestations of the syndrome and its insidious onset hamper its diagnosis. Besides the above symptoms, some objective signs are measured to make the definitive diagnosis of SS, using: ocular tests, notably Schirmer's I test and/or the Rose Bengal score; labial salivary gland biopsy, for assessing focal sialadenitis; scintigraphy, sialography, or unstimulated salivary flow, for evaluation of salivary gland involvement; and tests to detect the presence of Ro/SSA and/or La/SSB autoantibodies in serum.

Chapter IV – In primary Sjögren's Syndrome (pSS), health-related quality of life (HRQoL) and sexual health are impaired and correlated.

HRQoL in pSS is similarly altered in respect to patients with not Sjogren Sicca Syndrome (nS-SS) (presenting ocular and oral dryness, with negative autoantibodies and lip biopsy).

As expected, in pSS and ns-SS, HRQoL is related to the involvement of salivary and lachrymal glands, causing mainly dryness. In pSS and nS-SS, HRQoL is associated with anxiety and fatigue and, only in pSS, with depression. Pain, muscle skeletal concerns, and lung involvement are other determinants of HRQoL in pSS.

In women with pSS and nS-SS, sex health and ability, similarly altered, are affected by gynecological concerns, such as vaginal and vulvar dryness, more than by muscle-skeletal symptoms and, importantly, are related to impaired HRQoL.

Chapter V – Primary Sjögren's syndrome (pSS) (or Sjögren's syndrome) is a chronic autoimmune inflammatory disease characterized primarily by involvement of the exocrine glands. Multiple organs may also be affected, causing a highly variable spectrum of clinical manifestations. Most patients have less severe extraglandular symptoms such as fatigue, polyarthralgia and diffuse myalgia, while others develop serious systemic impairments including pneumonitis, vasculitis, peripheral neuropathy, glomerulonephritis and lymphoma. The disease predominantly affects females, with a peak incidence between 40-60 years-old, and its prevalence in the general population is approximately 0.1-0.5%. The etiology is unknown, but the autoimmune nature of SS is supported by the production of multiple circulating autoantibodies, mainly anti-Ro/SSA and anti-La/SSB. Peripheral nervous system (PNS) involvement is a well-recognized injury in this disease, which affects 10-20% of pSS patients. It is characterized by peripheral symmetric axonal sensorimotor polyneuropathy or pure sensory neuropathy. Central nervous system (CNS) involvement in pSS, although uncommon (0.3-6%), may aggravate the patient's clinical condition and lead to motor and cognitive sequelae. Retrospective studies assessing CNS damage in pSS suggest that the neurological manifestations are highly heterogeneous.

In this chapter, the frequency, pathogenesis, clinical features, diagnosis, differential diagnosis and treatment of the central nervous system involvement in pSS are reviewed.

Chapter VI – Sjögren's syndrome, an autoimmune disease characterized by exocrine gland dysfunction leading to dry mouth and dry eye diseases, is typified by lymphoplasmacytic infiltrations and a progressive destruction of the salivary and lacrimal glands. Despite an ever-increasing focus on identifying the underlying etiology of Sjögren's syndrome, defining factors that initiate this autoimmune disease and mechanisms that develop the following exocrine gland dysfunction remain a mystery.

The original explanatory concept for the pathogenesis of Sjögren's syndrome proposed a specific, self-perpetuating, immune mediated loss of acinar and ductal cells as the principal cause of salivary gland dysfunction. Accordingly, apoptosis, fibrosis and atrophy of the salivary glands would represent consequences of salivary gland hypofunction.

In this chapter the authors highlight the possible involvement of *regenerating gene* (*Reg*) in regeneration and destruction of salivary gland acinar and ductal cells in Sjögren's syndrome. *Reg* gene was originally isolated as a gene specifically overexpressed in regenerating pancreatic islets and constitute a growth factor family (Reg family). *Reg* gene product (*Reg* protein) is important in the pathophysiology of various human inflammatory diseases such as diabetes, inflammatory bowel disease(s), and Sjögren's syndrome. The authors describe how the salivary gland dysfunction is initiated and maintained, and how it can be regenerated or progressed mediated by *Reg* gene and Reg protein. They also touch on recent aspects of potential molecular mechanisms underlying immune-mediated salivary gland dysfunction prior to glandular destruction and atrophy, resulting in the symptoms of dryness in Sjögren's syndrome.

In: Sjögren's Syndrome
Editor: Eduardo M. Hernandez

ISBN: 978-1-63117-859-7


*Chapter I*

# Omega 3 Fatty Acids and Primary Sjogren's Syndrome: Overview and Exploratory Investigation

***J. Wu,*[1] *B. Nazir,*[1] *D. A. Brand*[2,4] *and S. E. Carsons*[1,3,*]**

[1]Department of Medicine and [2]Office of Health Outcomes Research, Winthrop-University Hospital, Mineola, NY, US

[3]Department of Medicine and [4]Department of Preventative Medicine, Stony Brook University School of Medicine, Stony Brook NY, US

## Abstract

**Objective:** To describe the relationship between intake of omega-3 fatty acids (ω3) and symptom severity in patients with primary Sjogren's Syndrome.

**Methods:** This exploratory cross-sectional study recruited adult Sjogren's patients during routine office visits to a faculty rheumatology practice, when subjects provided data on their diet during the previous year, reported their current symptoms, and gave consent for investigators to review their medical records to ascertain prescribed therapy for

* Corresponding author: S.E. Carsons, M.D. Division of Rheumatology, Allergy and Immunology Winthrop-University Hospital Clinical Campus. Suite 410, 120 Mineola Blvd, Mineola NY 11501. scarsons@winthrop.org.

Sjogren's syndrome. Patients completed a previously validated semi-quantitative food-frequency questionnaire, and they reported symptom severity (ocular sicca, oral sicca and overall Sjogren's-related symptoms) on three separate visual analog scales ranging from 0 to 100 (lowest to highest severity). A standard nutritional table indicating the ω3 content of common foods was applied to the food frequency data to estimate average daily ω3 consumption. Spearman's correlation coefficient was used to test the relationship between ω3 intake and symptom severity in patients receiving secretagogue therapy (e.g., cevimeline or pilocarpine), as well as in untreated patients. The Kruskal-Wallis test was used to compare symptom severity in 3 groups: pharmacologically treated patients, untreated patients reporting high intake of ω3 (≥500mg/d), and untreated patients reporting low intake of ω3 (<500mg/d).

**Results:** Among the 30 study subjects, the average daily intake of ω3 was 495±780mg/d (mean±SD). The average ocular, oral, and overall symptom severity scores were 56±29, 61±31, and 60±29, respectively. None of the correlations between ω3 intake and symptom severity were statistically significant ($p<0.05$) in either pharmacologically treated patients (n=12) or untreated patients (n=18). The mean ocular severity scores were 56, 53, and 57 in treated patients, untreated high-intake patients (n=6), and untreated low-intake patients (n=12), respectively. The corresponding oral severity scores were 56, 49, and 72, and the overall severity scores were 55, 49, and 70. While none of the differences in symptom severity across the 3 groups were statistically significant, the results do suggest possible beneficial effects of high ω3 intake for oral and overall symptoms that are roughly equivalent to the benefits of secretagogue therapy.

**Conclusion:** This exploratory investigation suggests the possibility that high intake of ω3 may have a beneficial effect on symptoms in patients with primary Sjogren's Syndrome who are not receiving secretagogue therapy. A larger study is needed to confirm or reject this hypotheses. A confirmatory result would make it worth considering ω3 supplementation as an alternative to pharmacologic therapy.

# Introduction

Primary Sjogren's Syndrome (pSS) is an autoimmune disease characterized by lymphocytic infiltration of exocrine glands and mucosae. The ocular surface of both conjunctiva and lacrimal glands show T-cell infiltration and upregulation of immune activation. Thus, anti-inflammatory agents are believed to be helpful for alleviating symptoms in pSS. Topical anti-inflammatory treatment of patients with dry eyes produces a reduction of activated lymphocytes in the conjunctiva [1]. In addition, anti-inflammatory therapies can reduce the signs and symptoms of keratoconjunctivitis sicca. Topical corticosteroids and cyclosporine A have been shown to control ocular inflammation [2].

A genetic and viral etiology is probably the most common cause in various autoimmune disorders, but chronic changes in environmental factors, particularly dietary antigens and lipids, can modify immunological function and can trigger or accelerate the disease process [3].

One dietary factor that may have an influence in pSS is the essential fatty acid pathway. Essential fatty acid deficiency leads to atrophy of salivary and lacrimal glands [4]. Omega-6 fatty acids (ω6) and omega-3 fatty acids (ω3) are of interest in pSS due to their anti-inflammatory effects. However, production and breakdown of inflammatory metabolites is highly regulated, and it is unclear that changes in substrate due to consumption of ω3 or ω6 (from the diet or supplements) have major effects on these inflammatory pathways in humans.

Generally, ω6, especially arachidonic acid, are known for their pro-inflammatory effects [3]. Some ω6, however, such as gamma linolenic acid (GLA) and linoleic acid (LA), have anti-inflammatory properties. Unlike arachidonic acid, which leads to formation of 2-series prostaglandins and 4-series leukotrienes (2 substances with proinflammatory effects), GLA and LA results in the production of 1-series prostaglandins which have anti-inflammatory properties. In addition, GLA and LA cannot be converted to leukotrienes but can form a 15-hydroxyl derivative that blocks the transformation of arachidonic acid to the inflammatory leukotrienes [5]. The metabolism of ω3 and ω6 to their anti- and pro- inflammatory molecules is shown in Figure 1. GLA and LA have been reported to have beneficial effects in the treatment of chronic inflammatory disorders, such as rheumatoid arthritis and pSS [1]. In one randomized, double-blind trial, primary Sjogren's patients had a significant improvement of ocular symptoms when treated with a mixture of GLA and LA for 8 weeks [6].

Conversely, ω3 have not been studied extensively in pSS [1]. Given the positive findings of anti-inflammatory ω6, it is strange to see so few studies on ω3 in pSS. Studies showing inconclusive results of ω3 on anti-inflammatory pathways and in other autoimmune diseases may be one reason. Fish oil supplementation in controlled studies does appear to inhibit production of cytokines, including interleukin-1 beta and tumor necrosis factor-alpha [7]. To achieve these effects, however, relatively high doses (>2 g /day) of fish oil may be necessary. It is not clear that a lower dose can produce the same substantial anti-inflammatory effects. Some recent studies on ω3 in pSS have shown promise. A recent cross-sectional study done using a food-frequency questionnaire found a higher dietary intake of ω3 is associated with a decreased incidence of dry eye syndrome in women [8]. Another study done using a similar food-frequency questionaire showed lower intake of polyunsaturated fat, linoleic acid, ω3, and other unsaturated fatty acids in women with pSS [9]. Although these were positive, another pilot study did not reveal significant beneficial effects on dry mouth with ω3 supplementation compared to controls [10].

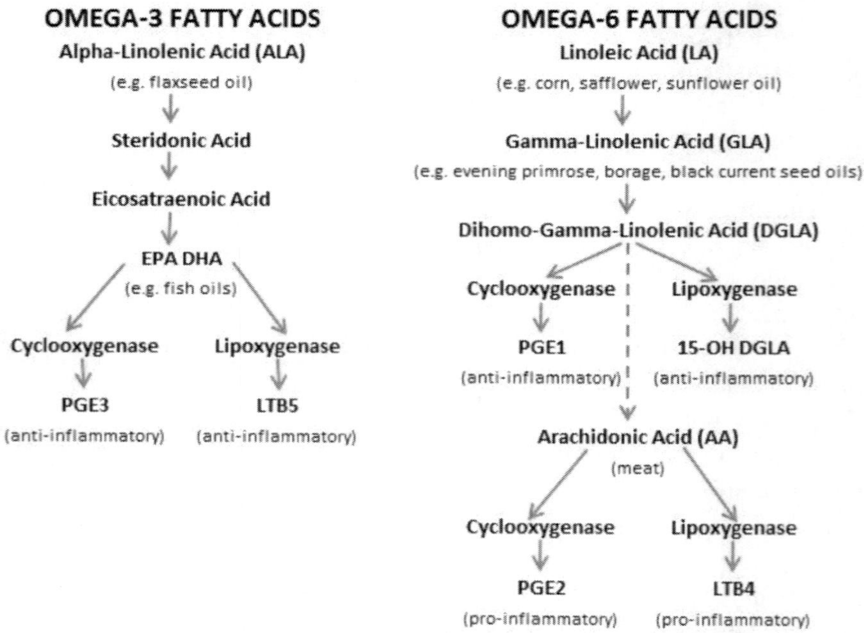


Figure 1. Metabolism of Omega-3 and Omega-6 Fatty Acids to their anti- and pro-inflammatory substrates. Examples of dietary sources of each essential fatty acid are displayed underneath the acid. Underneath each substrate is if they are anti- or pro-inflammatory. EPA, Eicosapentaenoic Acid; DHA, Docosahexaenoic Acid; PGE3, Series-3 Prostaglandins; LTB5, Leukotriene B5; PGE1, Series-1 Prostaglandins; LTB4, LEukotriene B4; 15-OH DGLA, 15-Hydroxydihomo-gamma-linolenic acid; PGE2, Series-2 Prostaglandins.

To our knowledge, there are no studies that assessed total ω3 and severity of symptoms in pSS. In our study, therefore, we assessed clinical symptoms and estimated total intake of ω3 in patients with pSS to evaluate a possible relationship. We hypothesized that higher intake of ω3 would be associated with less severe symptoms.

# Methods

## Study Design and Patients

This exploratory cross-sectional study recruited adult Sjogren's patients (ages 18-85 years) during routine office visits to a faculty rheumatology practice. Patients meeting the American-European Classification Criteria for primary Sjogren's Syndrome who gave consent to participate in the study were asked to describe their diet during the previous year, report their current symptoms, and allow investigators to review their medical records to ascertain prescribed therapy for Sjogren's syndrome. Patients were excluded if they had a malabsorption disorder (e.g., Celiac's disease, inflammatory bowel disease), were taking medications affecting absorption (e.g., cholestyramine, Orlistat), or had undergone a surgical procedure that could affect absorption (e.g., gastric bypass).

## Data Collection

### *Dietary Omega-3 Intake*

Subjects completed a validated semi-quantitative food-frequency questionnaire covering 120 commonly consumed foods [11]. For each food, the questionnaire specified a portion size, asked how often on average the subject had consumed that amount over the past year, and offered 9 choices ranging from "never" to "6x a day." We calculated the total intake of ω3 from seafood by assigning grams (g) of ω3 per serving as follows: 1.51 g for dark-flesh fish, 0.42 g for canned tuna fish, 0.48 g for light-flesh fish, and 0.32 g for shrimp, lobster, or scallops. These values were derived by weighting the mean values of ω3 reported for the most common types of fish caught in the United States [8]. While seafood is the main source of ω3 in the typical North American diet, we also estimated intake of ω3 from other sources such as plants and dietary supplements to yield a subject's total ω3 intake.

### *Symptom Severity*

Subjects reported symptom severity (ocular sicca, oral sicca and overall Sjogren's-related symptoms) on three separate visual analog scales that yielded scores ranging from 0 to 100 (lowest to highest severity). In addition, subjects were asked if they had extra glandular manifestations including joint pain, fatigue, cough, Raynaud's, rash, and neuropathic pain.

### Statistical Analysis

Spearman's correlation coefficient was used to test the relationship between ω3 intake and symptom severity in patients receiving secretagogue therapy (e.g., cevimeline or pilocarpine), and separately in untreated patients. The Kruskal-Wallis test was used to compare symptom severity in 3 groups: pharmacologically treated patients, untreated patients reporting high intake of ω3 (≥500mg/d), and untreated patients reporting low intake of ω3 (<500mg/d).

## Results

A total of 30 patients were enrolled in the study. No patient had to be excluded because of a malabsorption disorder or a medication or previous surgical procedure that could affect absorption.

The average daily intake of ω3 was 495±767mg/d (mean±SD), or 153±300mg/day excluding supplemention. (A total of 8 subjects reported taking ω3 supplements.) The average ocular, oral, and overall symptom severity scores were 56±28, 61±30, and 60±29, respectively. None of the correlations between ω3 intake and symptom severity were statistically significant ($p<0.05$) in either pharmacologically treated patients (n=12) or untreated patients (n=18). The mean ocular severity scores were 56, 53, and 57 in treated patients, untreated high-intake patients (n=6), and untreated low-intake patients (n=12), respectively. The corresponding oral severity scores were 55, 49, and 72, and the overall severity scores were 55, 49, and 70 (Figure 2). While none of the differences in symptom severity across the 3 groups were statistically significant, the results do suggest possible beneficial effects of high ω3 intake for oral and overall symptoms that appear to be roughly equivalent to the benefits of secretagogue therapy.

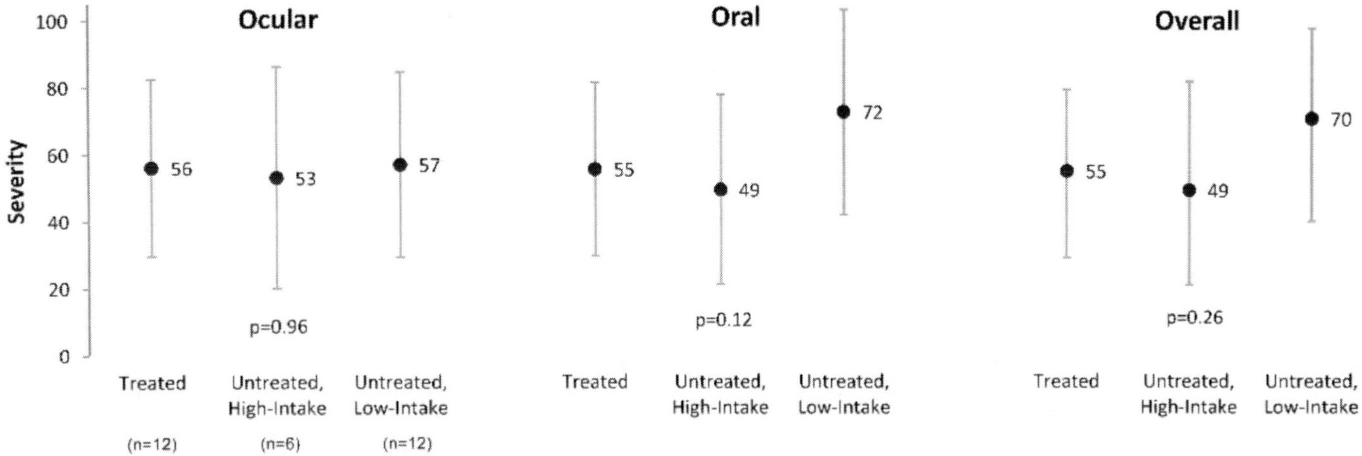


Figure 2. Severity of ocular, oral, and overall symptoms by treatment status and omega-3 intake. Each graph compares the mean symptom severity score reported by patients in one of three catetgories: (1) treated with a secretagogue, (2) untreated and reporting high intake of ω3 (≥500mg/d), and (3) untreated and reporting a low intake of ω3 (<500mg/d). On the symptom severity scale, 0 and 100 represent least and most severe, respectively. Error bars indicate standard deviations, and p-values refer to the comparison of mean scores among the three patient categories.

# Discussion

Sjogren's syndrome is an autoimmune disorder affecting 1% of the population. Most report severe ocular and oral dryness, glandular swelling, and fatigue. Treatment of pSS is usually symptomatic and therefore lubricating ophthalmic drops and sugar free candies to stimulate saliva are common options. Muscarinic agonists such as cevimeline and pilocarpine are two forms of pharmacologic therapies in use for sicca symptoms. Unfortunately, patients commonly complain of hyperhidrosis, sialorrhea, and other adverse reactions with use of these medications. Therefore, much needed alternative therapy is in demand. ω3 have gained interest due to their anti-inflammatory properties. In this investigation, we explored if ω3 have any effect on symptom severity in pSS. Our hypothesis was that a higher ω3 intake might alleviate severity of pSS symptoms through pathways involving anti-inflammatory lipids.

Although this exploratory study based on a small sample of Sjogren's patients did not demonstrate statistically significant benefits of dietary ω3 on pSS symptoms, the results do suggest that high ω3 intake may reduce the severity of oral dryness and global discomfort. These findings are consistent with the hypothesis that inflammation may have a central role in decreasing exocrine gland function in pSS.

The study depended on subjects' recall of dietary data. Although the nutritional survey is a well-validated instrument for assessing dietary intake, a subject's recall may be exaggerated in certain circumstances [11]. Since patients completed the survey in a doctor's office prior to their scheduled encounter with the physician, it is possible that the patient exaggerated answers to appear to be pursuing a healthier lifestyle. In this study, we also did not account for the effects of potential confounders such as lifestyle and comorbidity factors (e.g., exercise, smoking, diabetes, age).

The role of prostaglandins (PGs) in the pathogenesis of pSS is not well understood. PGs are divided into 3 different series [12]. Series 1 and 2 PGs are produced from ω6 while series 3 PGs are produced from ω3, which are believed to be less inflammatory. Case controlled studies have shown series 1 PGs (such as PGE1), produced from GLA and LA, can alleviate severity of pSS symptoms while the series 2 PGs (such as PGE2 and PGF2) produced from arachidonic acid increased severity of pSS symptoms [1, 6, 13]. Although series 3 PGs (such as PGE3 and PGI3) produced from ω3 [12] are known for their anti-inflammatory properties, as of this time, the authors are unaware of any studies demonstrating the effect of these specific PGs in pSS. Thus, the effects of dietary fat on the immune system are extremely complex and lymphocyte function can be modulated in several ways with ω3 possibly only playing a limited role [14]. The ratio between ω6 and ω3 may be just as or more important than the total intake of ω3. The recommended ω6 to ω3 ratio is about 4:1, however, a typical American diet consists of a ratio closer to 12-16:1 [8]. A more extensive study examining the actual ω6 to ω3 ratio in pSS may be of interest.

One of the primary goals in our study was to examine total ω3 intake (dietary and/or supplemental) as well as the use of current pharmacologic therapy in pSS. We classified subjects with ω3 >500mg per day as high ω3 intake because this value is the current recommended intake for dietary health set by the United States Department of Agriculture in the Dietary Guidelines for Americans in 2005 [14]. The average dietary ω3 intake in our study was 153mg/day. This appears to be significantly lower than the 370 mg daily dietary ω3 intake in control subjects reported by Cermak et al. in their nutritional study of Sjogren's and control subjects. In Cermak et al's study, the average dietary ω3 intake in their pSS subjects were 230mg/day which was consistent with but slightly higher than what we report here. In either case, both groups of pSS subjects had lower dietary ω3 intake than the control group reported by Cermack [9]. It is not clear why we see this result since there is no evidence to suggest that a lower dietary ω3 intake is associated with the development of Sjogren's syndrome. It is perhaps more likely that the sicca symptoms may result in lower fish intake. Although it was not specifically included in our survey, a few subjects did inform us that they did not consume fish because fish and/or other seafood left an unpalatable taste due to the severe oral dryness.

In total, 27% of our study subjects took omega 3 supplementation. This is slightly below the national average of Americans who reported having tried ω3 supplementation according to the 2007 National Health Interview Survey. In that survey, 37% (10.9 million) of adult Americans reported using an ω3 supplement for health reasons [15]. Since there is no current evidence that ω3 supplementation is beneficial in pSS, it is reasonable that a lesser amount of people are taking ω3 supplements in a pSS population compared to the average population who is likely taking ω3 supplements for confirmed health benefits such as cardiovascular disease. However, it appears that pSS patients are consuming less dietary ω3 intake than the average population, possibly due to oral discomfort secondary to sicca symptoms. This may be a population that should be targeted for dietary ω3 supplementation especially if future data demonstrates a significant benefit in improvement of sicca complaints.

This exploratory investigation suggests the possibility that high intake of ω3 may have a beneficial effect on symptoms in patients with primary Sjogren's Syndrome who are not receiving secretagogue therapy. A larger study is needed to confirm or reject this hypotheses. A confirmatory result would make it worth considering ω3 supplementation as an alternative or adjunct to pharmacologic therapy.

# References

[1] Aragona, P; Bucolo, C; et al. Systemic omega-6 essential fatty acid treatment and PGE1 tear content in sjogren's syndorme patients. *Invest. Ophthalmol. Vis. Sci. 2005*; 46(12):4474-4479.

[2] Pflugfelder, SC. Antiinflammatory therapy for dry eye. *Am. J. Ophthalmol.* 2004; 137:337-342.

[3] Fernandes, G. Dietary lipids and risk of autoimmune disease. *Clin Immunol Immunopathol.* 1994; 72(2):193-197.

[4] Horrobin, DF. Essential fatty acid and prostaglandin metabolism in sjogren's syndrome, systemic sclerosis, and rheumatoid arthritis. *Scand J Rheumatol.* 1986; 61(suppl):242-245.

[5] Belch, JJ and Hill, A. Evening primrose oil and borage oil in rheumatologic conditions. *Am J Clin Nutr.* 2000; 71(suppl):352S-356S.

[6] Oxholm, P; Manthorpe, R; et al. Patients with primary sjogren's syndrome treated for two months with evening primrose oil. *Scand J Rheumatol.* 1986; 15:103-108.

[7] James, MJ; Gibson RA, et al. Dietary polyunsaturated fatty acids and inflammatory mediator production. *Am J Clin Nutr.* 2000; 71:343S.

[8] Miljanovic, B; Trivedi, KA; et al. Relation between dietary n-3 and n-6 fatty acids and clinically diagnosed dry eye syndrome in women. *Am J Clin Nutr.* 2005; 82:887-893.

[9] Cermak, JM; Papas, AS; et al. Nutrient intake in women with primary and secondary sjogren's syndrome. *Eur J Clin Nutr.* 2003; 57:328-334.

[10] Singh, M; Stark, PC; et al. Effect of omega-3 and vitamin E supplementation on dry mouth in patients with Sjögren's syndrome. *Spec Care Dentist.* 2010; 30(6):225-9.

[11] Willett, W. *Nutritional epidemiology.* 2nd ed. New York, NY: Oxford University Press, 1998.

[12] Bagga, D; Wang, L; et al. Differential effects of prostaglandin derived from ω-6 and ω-3 polyunsaturated fatty acids on COX-2 expression and IL-6 secretion. *PNAS.* 2003; 100(4):1751-1756.

[13] Macri, A; Gluffrida, S; et al. Effect of linoleic acid and gamma-linolenic acid on tear production, tear clearance and on the ocular surface after photorefractive keratectomy. *Graefes Arch Clin Exp Ophthalmol.* 2003; 241(7):561-566.

[14] Gebauer, SK; Psota, TL; et al. n−3 Fatty acid dietary recommendations and food sources to achieve essentiality and cardiovascular benefits. Am J Clin Nutr. 2006; 83(6) S1526-1535S.

[15] Barnes, PM; Bloom, B. Complementary and alternative medicine use among adults and children: United States, 2007. *National Health Statistics Reports.* 2008; 12:1-24.

In: Sjögren's Syndrome
Editor: Eduardo M. Hernandez

ISBN: 978-1-63117-859-7


*Chapter II*

# An Overview of the Clinical Manifestations and Management of Primary Sjögren's Syndrome

***Josephine Vila[1*], Rebecca Batten[2,*] and Wan-Fai Ng[1,2,†]***
[1]Newcastle upon Tyne Hospitals NHS Foundation Trust
[2]Musculoskeletal Research Group, Institute of Cellular Medicine, Newcastle University, UK

## Abstract

Primary Sjögren's syndrome (PSS) is a multi-system, immune-mediated, condition of unknown aetiology characterized by dryness of the eyes and mouth, pain and disabling fatigue. Other organs such as the skin, the nervous system, the lungs and the kidneys can also be affected. PSS is also associated with a markedly increased risk of lymphoma development. The health-related quality of life of patients with PSS is significantly impaired and the direct and indirect health economic cost associated with the condition is substantial.

* Contributed equally to the chapter.
† Corresponding author: Wan-Fai Ng, Musculoskeletal Research Group, Institute of Cellular Medicine, Newcastle University, Newcastle upon Tyne, NE2 4HH, United Kingdom, e-mail: Wan-Fai.Ng@ncl.ac.uk.

The true prevalence of PSS is unknown but is estimated to be between 0.1-0.4% of the adult population with a strong female bias. The diagnosis is often delayed with PSS patients presenting to their doctors after suffering from the symptoms for many years. Improved links between rheumatologists, ophthalmologists, oral medicine specialists, dentists, opticians, and general practitioners can facilitate early diagnosis and reduce risk of long-term disability.

The American European Consensus Group (AECG) classification criteria 2002 are the current gold standard for the classification of PSS, although provisional American College of Rheumatology (ACR) criteria have recently been published. The development of consensus criteria by the ACR-European League Against Rheumatism (EULAR) working group to bring together the two criteria is in progress. Additionally, salivary gland ultrasound may also be an important component of the diagnostic criteria in the near future. Salivary gland sialometry, sialochemistry, tear osmolarity may be useful adjuncts, and the discovery of new diagnostic biomarkers is an area of active research.

Optimal assessment of patients with PSS, should encompass not only objective parameters such as abnormalities in blood tests and changes in tear and salivary flow, but also patient-reported outcome measures and impact on quality of life. Symptoms of PSS are often non-specific, therefore these symptoms must be actively explored. The recent development of EULAR outcome measurement tools for the assessment of systemic disease activity and patient-reported outcome has greatly facilitated standardised assessment of PSS in clinics and in research.

Management of PSS can be broadly classified into interventions targeting the glandular or systemic manifestations of the disease. Evidence-based strategies in PSS management remain elusive, instead, treatments are often based on empirical evidence or experience of the treating clinicians. The effective management of fatigue remains a major challenge. Recent advances in the understanding of PSS pathogenesis have led to the study of several biological therapies for the PSS with some encouraging data. Finally, optimal management of patients with PSS requires expertise from different disciplines such as ophthalmology, oral medicine and restorative dentistry.

## Introduction and Classification

Sjögren's syndrome can be encountered alone (primary Sjögren's syndrome (PSS)), or in the presence of other rheumatic diseases (secondary Sjögren's syndrome). The condition is named after Henrik Sjögren, a Swedish ophthalmologist, who described it in his doctorate thesis, published in 1933

[1]. He used the term 'keratoconjunctivitis sicca' to specifically distinguish the ocular surface features from those seen in vitamin-A deficiency (xerophthalmia). The clinical and histological features were described as early as 1892 in a patient with parotid gland swelling [2] by Jan Mikulicz-Radecki, an Austro-Polish surgeon. This chapter will focus on PSS unless otherwise stated and will describe the clinical features, diagnostic methods, and management of this condition.

PSS is a chronic, immune-mediated, multisystem disease of unknown aetiology characterized by focal lymphocytic infiltration of exocrine glands associated with dry mouth and eyes, pain and disabling fatigue. The prevalence and health economic impact are comparable with rheumatoid arthritis (RA). However, PSS research to date has been comparatively poorly supported [3]. Multisystem involvement can also affect the joints, lung, skin and peripheral nervous system [4]. Cytopenias, hypocomplementaemia and cryoglobulinaemia can occur and if present, confer a worse prognosis.

## Epidemiology

The true prevalence of PSS is unknown but is estimated to affect between 0.1-0.4% of the adult population with no known ethnic preponderance. The female to male ratio is traditionally reported as 9:1 but possibly as high as 13:1 [5] PSS can affect any age group, including children. It typically presents in the fifth or sixth decade of life, although the disease process may have started many years before.

## Clinical Features

### *Ocular Manifestations*

#### **Dry Eye**

The causes of dry eye in PSS are multifactorial and can arise due to defects of tears and the ocular surface resulting in symptoms of discomfort, visual disturbance, and tear film instability with potential damage to the ocular surface [6]. Ocular surface inflammation follows with increased tear film osmolarity. Dry eye occurs principally as a result of abnormalities of the lacrimal functional unit, which represents an integrated system consisting of the lacrimal glands, the ocular surface (cornea, conjunctiva), eyelids and meibomian glands (MG) together with the sensory-motor nerves that connect them [7].

The surface of the eye is coated with a tear film, which performs the essential functions of immunological defence of the eye, lubrication and nutrition. The tear film consists of a superficial aqueous phase secreted by the lacrimal gland which supports epithelial cell growth and function. Homeostasis of the tear film involves complex hormonal and neuronal regulatory mechanisms [8]. Underneath the tear film, is a hydrophilic mucinous layer synthesised by conjunctival goblet cells that limits adhesion of pathogens or foreign bodies to the surface of the eye [9]. The meibomian glands (MG) secrete the lipids which make up the most superficial layer in association with aqueous proteins, which provide further barrier function, minimise evaporation and confer tear film stability. The cornea is avascular and is supplied with oxygen and nutrients by the muco-aqueous gradient between these two layers. The cornea, lacrimal glands, goblet cells, and MG are all richly innervated with parasympathetic, sympathetic and sensory nerves which have complex stimulatory or inhibitory roles. Abnormalities can result in dysregulation of lacrimal function [10]. Known contributing factors include tear film hyperosmolarity, reduced tear mucins and lipids, increased tear film break-up and reduced tear volume causing increased shear-stresses between the lids and globe. Autoimmune damage and destruction of the lacrimal glands causes the release of inflammatory mediators into the tear film [11] which stimulates a cascade of signalling pathways and the production of inflammatory cytokines to produce a self-perpetuating autoimmune response [12]. Chronic dryness of the ocular surface leads to further inflammation and lacrimal gland and conjunctival epithelium destruction. Once dry eye disease has been established, self perpetuating inflammation is the key mechanism of ocular surface injury resulting in hypersensitivity of the nociceptive sensory nerves, neural activation and symptomatology. Secondary loss of lipid layer due to MG obstruction, stagnation, dysfunction and eventual destruction (with or without associated Staphylococcal colonisation and/or hypersensitivity) further compounds ocular surface inflammation.

PSS patients may report a range of ocular symptoms including foreign body sensation, ocular fatigue, painful, dry, gritty, or burning eyes which can vary in severity from mild discomfort to severe constant pain with associated visual disturbances. Photophobia is common. However, this symptom can be the presenting feature of uveitis which, though rare in PSS, is a potentially debilitating complication and can be treated with topical or systemic steroids.

In some patients, symptoms exceed clinical signs presumably due to nociceptive sensory receptor hypersensitivity [13].

### *Oral Manifestations*

#### Xerostomia

Xerostomia or dry mouth is the major oral symptom of Sjögren's syndrome and can have a significant adverse effect on quality of life [14]. Patients may describe the effects dry mouth in many ways:

- Difficulty eating dry food eg crackers
- The tongue or food sticking to the roof of the mouth
- Needing to drink water through the night
- Difficulty speaking or hoarse voice
- Mouth pain due to oral candidiasis, periodontal disease and angular chelitis
- Altered taste perception
- Difficulty swallowing (dysphagia)
- Halitosis
- Poor denture retention or increased dental caries

Loss of salivary gland function is already prominent in the early stages of disease and is associated with difficulty chewing and swallowing food. The submandibular and sublingual glands are normally active at rest, therefore patients commonly report xerostomia at rest and at night in the early stages. The parotid glands, which secrete saliva when stimulated, tend to be affected late [15]. Hyposalivation is also associated with difficulty with speech, oral discomfort due to ulceration and fissures, reduced taste sensation and sensitivity to coarse or spicy foods.

Patients with advanced xerostomia may exhibit a dry oral mucosa, cracked, atrophic lips and a pale, smooth tongue with loss of dorsal papillae and fissuring. The parotid duct, when visualised, can be narrowed and the sublingual salivary pool decreased. Marked dental caries are common. Patients are also susceptible to oral infections, particularly oral candidiasis (which may present simply as 'sore mouth' rather than classical visible white plaques) and angular chelitis (fungal infection at the corners of the mouth).

*Salivary Gland Swelling*

Chronic or intermittent salivary gland swelling is common, affecting up to 2/3 of all patients with PSS. It can be unilateral or bilateral and is thought to be a result of the generalised autoimmune inflammatory response. Lymphoma, which presents with painless nodular lymphadenopathy should be excluded as it is 16 times more common in PSS patients than in the general population [16].

In younger patients or children the presenting feature is commonly painless swelling of the parotid and/or submandibular salivary glands.

*Extra-Glandular Manifestations*

### Constitutional

Symptoms of anorexia, weight loss, fevers, night sweats and fatigue are frequently experienced and may profoundly limit patient activity.

### Articular & Muscular

Articular manifestations occur in between 30-60% of patients with PSS [17]. Arthritis is polyarticular, peripheral and symmetrical. It is usually non-deforming and non-erosive, affecting the metacarpal phalangeal (MCP), proximal interphalangeal (PIP) joints and wrists. Synovitis is generally mild, however, the presence of joint involvement is a predictor for other systemic involvement.

Myalgia and weakness are common symptoms in PSS but clinically significant myositis is relatively rare.

### Respiratory

Drying of mucous membranes predisposes patients to a chronic dry cough and hoarseness is common in PSS. Significant lung pathology occurs relatively infrequently. There is diversity in the reported prevalence of lung disease, probably due to the lack of universal classification criteria. Pulmonary function abnormalities are found in up to 25% of patients. One study found a population-based prevalence of clinical pulmonary involvement of 22% among patients with PSS [18]. These patients had reduced quality of life (QoL) and a 4-fold increase in 10 year mortality. Abnormal high resolution computer tomography scans (HRCT) were found in 50 patients (23%) and abnormal pulmonary function (PFTs) in 34 patients (16%). Ground glass attenuation is the most common HRCT abnormality (64.3%) [19]. Lower lobe bronchiectasis, reticular changes and honeycombing can also occur. A recent study of 522 patients [20] demonstrated that 23.2% had interstitial lung disease, 12.5% pulmonary artery hypertension, 9.2% multiple pulmonary bullae, 6% pleural effusions and 5.6% pulmonary nodules.

Non-specific interstitial pneumonia is the most common type of interstitial lung disease in PSS. Patients may present with chronic dry cough, breathlessness on exertion or constrictive defects on PFT's. Histopathology characteristically demonstrates diffuse thickening of the alveolar septae and lymphocytic infiltration [21]. Lymphocytic interstitial pneumonitis (LIP) is a rare but well recognized condition associated with PSS. The presentation is acute with fever, cough, and dyspnoea, with bibasilar pulmonary infiltrates. LIP usually responds well to treatment with steroids. The main differential diagnosis is infection [22, 23].

Airways abnormalities such as bronchiolitis or bronchiectasis can occur as a result of chronic inflammation and lymphoplasmacytic infiltration of central and peripheral bronchi and bronchioles.

A study of possible predictive parameters found that male/female ratio, mean age and unsurprisingly, smoking was higher in patients with lung involvement. The presence of hypergammaglobulinaemia, lymphopenia, RF and anti-Ro and anti-La had a high specificity but low sensitivity to detect PSS associated lung disease.

## Neurological

There is a broad spectrum of neurological manifestations of PSS. Peripheral neuropathy affects up to 25% of patients. The types of peripheral neuropathies depend on the fibres involved. Pure sensory neuropathy presents, most commonly, as painful dysaesthesia due to degeneration of cutaneous axons and may be diagnosed by skin biopsy. It can also manifest as sensory ataxia or distal symmetric sensory loss [24]. In sensorimotor polyneuropathy the sensory and motor axons are affected, the onset is generally insidious and it may affect up to 25% of patients with PSS [25]. Mononeuropathy and mononeuritis multiplex classically affects the lateral popliteal nerve and presents with foot drop. It is associated with cryoglobulinaemic vasculitis.

Autoimmune demyelinating neuropathy can present, like multiple sclerosis, with paraplegia, sensory change and urinary retention, white matter changes on magnetic resonance imaging (MRI) and matched oligoclonal bands in cerebrospinal fluid and serum [26]. Severe central nervous system (CNS) involvement is uncommon.

Many PSS patients have autonomic dysfunction [27-29], for example postural hypotension and dizziness, urinary retention, abnormal sweating and nocturnal diarrhoea. These symptoms were found to correlate with systemic disease activity and overall symptom burden in a large PSS cohort [30].

## Cutaneous

Cutaneous involvement is a well-recognised extra-glandular feature of PSS. It includes Raynaud's phenomenon, pruritus, dry skin, photosensitivity, cutaneous lesions similar to those seen in lupus (suggesting overlap of disease related anti-Ro), purpuric vasculitis (more common when anti-Ro and anti-La are positive and with hypergammaglobulinaemia), erythema nodosum, livido reticularis, lichen planus, vitiligo, cutaneous amyloidosis, annular granuloma, and granulomatous panniculitis. Cutaneous vasculitis is recognised in up to 10% of PSS patients and is associated with increased morbidity and a worse prognosis. In most cases it is a mild, self-limiting condition but can occasionally be persistent and severe. Small vessel vasculitis (leucocytoclastic vasculitis), which is the predominant type, manifests as palpable purpura, urticarial lesions or erythematous maculopapules. Systemic involvement occurs in 44% of patients with small vessel vasculitis in association with cryoglobulins in 30% of these [31]. Patients with cutaneous vasculitis have a higher prevalence of other extra-glandular and immunological features of PSS. Hypergammaglobulinaemic purpura causes a non-palpable purpura usually on the lower legs [31]. Histology with immunoflourescence demonstrates immune complex deposition. Subacute cutaneous lupus is a photosensitive, non-scarring rash, usually on the face, arms and front of the chest.

Raynaud's phenomenon affects up to 80% of patients with PSS [32]. The prevalence in one large study was 13% and in half of these patients, Raynaud's phenomenon was the presenting symptom of PSS [33].

### *Genitourinary and Kidneys*

Symptoms of urinary dysfunction are common. Walker et al. [34] found self reported severe urological symptoms in 61% of patients with PSS compared to 40% of controls with osteoarthritis (OA). The difference was predominantly in symptoms which could be attributable to bladder irritability associated with urgency. These symptoms are due to disturbances of muscarinic receptors and are possibly mediated by muscarinic receptor antibodies. Recurrent urinary tract infections affect 30% of patients with RA with secondary Sjögren's syndrome compared to 6% of patients with RA alone [35]. Habitual leucocyturia was also more common in patients with secondary Sjögren's syndrome. Chronic interstitial cystitis is often seen in association with connective tissue diseases. 90% of sufferers are female. The presence of this condition is suggested by recurrent dysuria in the absence of bacterial infection, and the diagnosis confirmed by cystoscopy and biopsy. The symptoms are often exacerbated in PSS patients due to the increased fluid intake to alleviate oral dryness.

Clinically significant renal disease is rare in PSS and most of the available evidence comes from case series. Approximately 5% of patients with PSS develop clinically significant renal involvement [36]. The overall 5-year survival rate in one series of patients with renal involvement is 85%, statistically significantly reduced compared to those without. A third of patients with renal involvement go on to develop chronic renal failure. Mild proteinuria is common, 44% of patients in one series had proteinuria of 1.5 – 0.42 g/24h. Renal complications include interstitial nephritis due to lymphocytic infiltration and leading to renal tubular acidosis. Patients may present with osteomalacia, renal stones, nephrocalcinosis or rarely hypokalaemic paralysis. Patients with renal tubular acidosis tend to have longer disease durations and are more likely to have proteinuria, hypertension and raised creatinine than those without. Glomerulonephritis, mediated by immune complex deposition in the context of systemic vasculitis, is associated with cryoglobulinaemia, hypocomplementaemia and increased risk of lymphoma. It presents later in the course of the disease and has been associated with increased morbidity and mortality.

Vaginal dryness is a common symptom, affecting 3 out of 4 women with PSS compared to 5% of the general population [37]. This can lead to dyspareunia and recurrent urinary tract infection [35]. Sexual dysfunction is a symptom, rarely volunteered during a medical consultation unless specifically sought. PSS patients are also susceptible to vulval and vaginal infections.

### *Gastrointestinal and Liver*

Dysphagia is common in PSS. Patients may present with reflux and it is important to identify and treat Helicobacter Pylori infection in these patients as it has been associated with the development of MALT lymphoma. PSS has been reported in up to 15% of patients with biopsy proven coeliac disease [38]. Antibodies to tissue transglutamase are found in up to 12% of PSS cases and the majority of these have confirmed coeliac disease. Patients may also present with diarrhoea or constipation as a result of autonomic dysfunction.

A link between sicca symptoms and primary biliary cirrhosis (PBC) has been demonstrated. A significant number of patients with PBC suffer from sicca symptoms. Anti-Ro/La are present in up to 50% of patients with PBC

[39]. Anti-mitochondrial antibody (AMA) and associated PBC is found in up to 5% of PSS patients. Autoimmune hepatitis can also occur in PSS [40, 41].

Over a third of PSS patients have a mild elevation of pancreatic enzymes [42] but clinically significant pancreatic involvement occurs in no more than 1%.

### *Haematological / Immunological*

Haematological and immunological manifestations of PSS are commonly asymptomatic. Mild autoimmune cytopenias, hypocomplementaemia, a positive rheumatoid factor (RF) or antinuclear antibody (ANA), raised acute phase reactants and hypergammaglobulinaemias are common reasons for referral as they are increasingly tested in primary care [41].

Anaemia occurs in up to a third of PSS patients [43]. Causes include anaemia of chronic disease (69% of anaemic patients), autoimmune haemolytic anaemia (18%) and iron deficiency anaemia (9%). Leucopenia occurs in 15% and thrombocytopenia in 11% of cases of PSS.

Hypocomplementaemia is associated with cryoglobulinaemia and leucopenia. Low C4 is an independent risk factor for the development of vasculitis [44] and low C4 and /or C3 an independent risk factor for B-cell lymphoma. Hypergammaglobulinaema, found in the majority of the patients positive for anti-Ro/La, is another marker of severity of PSS with more aggressive disease and extra-glandular manifestations [45, 46].

### *Autoantibodies*

Anti-Ro (SSA) and anti-La (SSB) are the most commonly occurring and identified (as part of the extractable nuclear antigen [ENA] screen) autoantibodies in PSS. Approximately two-thirds of patients with PSS have anti-Ro antibodies and one-third have anti-La antibodies [47]. The presence of these antibodies in PSS is associated with more aggressive disease with earlier disease onset, longer duration, higher frequency of extra-glandular manifestations, more intense lymphocytic infiltration of the minor salivary glands and parotid gland enlargement [48]. Very few patients have anti-La antibodies in the absence of anti-Ro antibodies. It is possible that the initial autoantibody response is directed against the Ro antigen and then ‘spreads’ to involve the La antigen [49]. The presence of RF and ANA is also commonly seen in PSS (50-90% ANA positivity) but are not sensitive or specific for PSS. Several other autoantibodies have been identified in patients with PSS which are not routinely measured in clinical practice. Anti-alpha-fodrin IgG and IgA antibodies have been found to be useful diagnostic markers [50]. A number of studies have suggested that autoantibodies directed against the G-protein-coupled muscarinic acetylcholine receptor (M3R), found in exocrine cells are an important factor in the reduced secretory function in PSS [51]. There are, however, some conflicting reports in the literature [52]. Anti-carbonic anhydrase antibodies [53], anti-ICA69 antibodies [54] and anti-aquaporin antibodies [55, 56] have also been linked to PSS pathogenesis. A low titre of dsDNA antibody has been described in a small proportion (<5%) of the anti-Ro/La positive patients. ANA and RF may be positive at diagnosis but are not associated with higher disease activity scores.

### *Thyroid Disease*

Autoimmune thyroiditis is nine times more frequent in PSS than the general population and PSS is ten times more frequent in patients with autoimmune thyroid disease [57].

Therefore, a diagnosis of thyroid disease should be sought and excluded in patients with PSS and vice versa. 37% of patients with autoimmune thyroid disease have an objectively dry mouth and 23% have objectively dry eyes [58]. Hypothyroidism is the most common autoimmune disease developed by PSS patients during follow-up of 10.5 years, with subclinical hypothyroidism the most common hormonal pattern [20%]. Antigens are shared by both thyroid and salivary glands, which could be responsible for the association between the two diseases. Immunogenetic studies had suggested that they have shared genetic predisposition.

### *Fatigue*

Up to 70% of patients suffer with fatigue. The mechanism is poorly understood, but is thought to be part of the systemic inflammatory response, although other non-biological factors may also contribute. It is associated with poor health-related quality of life and a major contributing factor to loss of work productivity in PSS patients.

### *Lymphoma*

PSS is associated with a markedly increased risk of development of Non-Hodgkin's Lymphoma (Standardised Incidence Risk [SIR] 18.8%) when compared the risk of lymphoma development in other autoimmune diseases, such as SLE (SIR 7.5% – moderate risk), and RA (SIR 3.3% - low risk). The prevalence of lymphoma increases from 3.4% in the first 5 years to 9-9.8% at 15 years [16, 59]. The majority of lymphomas are of the mucosa-associated lymphoid tissue (MALT), B-cell type. The classical presentation is of a unilateral, firm swelling in the parotid gland but it can occur elsewhere.

Chronic antigenic stimulation, present from the early stages of PSS results in polyclonal B-Cell activation. This in turn gives rise B-cell clones causing neoplasia. Risk factors for the development of lymphoma include: recurrent or persistent swelling of the salivary glands, lymphadenopathy, cryoglobulinaemia, splenomegaly, chronically low complement factors (C3, C4), lymphopenia, skin vasculitis, M-components in serum or urine, peripheral neuropathy, glomerulonephritis, elevated beta-2 microglobulin, $CD4^+$ T-lymphocytopenia, and germinal center-like structures in salivary gland biopsies. There are 2 recognised types of lymphoma in PSS:

1) Marginal Zone Lymphomas, of which there are 2 types:
   a) Extranodal marginal zone lymphomas (MALT lymphomas)
   b) Nodal marginal zone lymphomas
2) Aggressive lymphomas such as Diffuse Large B-Cell Lymphoma (DLBCL)

## PSS in Pregnancy

Pregnancy complications for patients with anti-Ro or anti-La include neonatal lupus, a serious complication of which is congenital AV heart block. Other complications of neonatal lupus in decreasing frequency include cutaneous, hepatobiliary, haematological, neurological, and splenic manifestations [60].

A neonatal lupus rash (usually appearing at 6 weeks of age, lasting 17 weeks with complete resolution in the vast majority) occurs in around 10-20% and other laboratory abnormalities in up to a third of babies born to anti-Ro/La positive mothers.

The majority of mothers are asymptomatic and diagnosed only with the birth of an affected child. The incidence of congenital heart block is estimated at 1-2% in women with anti-Ro, but increases to >20% in a mother with one previously affected child [60].

PSS has also been associated with an increased risk of spontaneous abortion and foetal loss [61]. Fertility seems not to be impaired. Recent studies suggest that pre-term delivery, low birth weight infants and caesarean section are more prevalent [62].

## Health-Related Quality of Life

PSS is associated with markedly impaired health-related quality of life (HR-QoL) [63-65]. Disease-specific instrument to evaluate HR-QoL in PSS have not yet been developed and validated. Therefore investigators have applied instruments such as Medical Outcomes Study Short form-36 (SF-36) [64-73] or Short Form-20 (SF-20), (74) WHOQoL-BREF [75] and Nottingham Health Profile [76] to assess HR-QoL in patients with PSS and have demonstrated that PSS patients experience substantially reduced HR-QoL comparable to other "rheumatic" conditions such as RA, SLE and fibromyalgia [3]. These studies also reported a diverse range of clinical and laboratory parameters that correlate with HR-QoL. Fatigue and psychological factors appear to play a more important role than dryness and objective laboratory measures. In a large PSS cohort in the UK [63], PSS patients were found to have significantly impaired EQ-5D utility values compared with the UK general population. Interestingly, the distribution of EQ-5D utility values exhibited a bi-modal distribution with some patients with no significant impairment to their HR-QoL, while the HR-QoL of some PSS patients was markedly reduced. EQ-5D utility values are significantly related to pain and depression scores in PSS. Fatigue, anxiety and body mass index are other predictors of EQ-5D utility values.

## Prognosis and Outcome

There is no overall increase in all-cause mortality in PSS compared with the general population. When subgroups of PSS are compared, there is an excess mortality associated with lymphoproliferative malignancy [77]. The strongest predictor for unfavourable outcome being low C3 and/or C4 levels at the time of diagnosis [78]. There is however, a significant adverse impact on the HR-QoL with substantial direct and indirect health economic costs. A recent study reported an indirect annual health care cost of £7677, compared with £892 for a healthy subject [79]. Employment rates are significantly lower, and the level of disability compensation claims significantly greater when compared to healthy subjects matched for age and gender [65]. This demonstrates a significant health and economic burden to patients and society, and should prompt timely investigation, diagnosis and management.

## Making a Diagnosis

There have been 12 different classification or diagnostic criteria published for Sjögren's syndrome since 1965 [80]. A number of these criteria were proposed in the 1980's resulting in major debate as to the relative merits of each [81].

The preliminary European criteria [82] were published in 1993 after collaboration between experts from 12 European countries. They included six components: symptoms of oral dryness (identified through the presence of at least one out of three 'dry mouth' questions) and similarly for dry eyes, objective eye dryness, objective oral dryness, a positive labial salivary gland biopsy (> 1 focus score/4mm$^2$) and positive anti-Ro/La antibodies. Four of the six components were required to make a diagnosis of PSS. Exclusion criteria were also proposed (hepatitis C infection, sarcoidosis, head and neck radiotherapy, acquired immunodeficiency syndrome, pre-existing lymphoma, graft-versus-host disease, use of anticholinergic drugs). These criteria were subsequently modified in 2002 to require the presence of either positive anti-Ro/La antibodies or positive labial salivary gland biopsy to form the American-European Consensus Group (AECG) criteria [83]. The diagnosis of PSS is also fulfilled if 3 out of the 4 objective criteria are present. Devised to ensure standardisation of the diagnosis of patients taking part in clinical trials, the AECG classification criteria is currently the most widely used criteria to guide diagnosis in clinical practice, although in reality other investigations are often required to rule out differential diagnoses [83].

**AECG (2002) Classification criteria**

For a diagnosis of Primary Sjögren's Syndrome, 4 out of 6 criteria must be met, and must include either IV (histopathology) or VI (autoantibodies).

I. *Ocular Symptoms* (dry eyes ≥ 3 months, foreign body sensation in eyes, use of artificial tears ≥ 3 times per day)
II. *Oral Symptoms* (dry mouth ≥ 3 months, recurrent or persistent swollen salivary glands, need for liquids to swallow dry foods)
III. *Ocular Signs* (Schirmer's ≤5mm/5 min, positive vital dye staining of eye surface)
IV. *Histopathology* (lymphocytic sialadenitis focal score ≥ 1 focus/4mm$^2$)

V. *Oral Signs* (Unstimulated whole saliva flow $\leq$ 1.5ml/15min, abnormal parotid sialography, abnormal salivary scintigraphy)
VI. *Autoantibodies* (anti-SSA/Ro or Anti-SSB/La or both)

Exclusion criteria: History of head and neck radiation, Hepatitis C infection, Acquired immunodeficiency syndrome, Sarcoidosis, Amyloidosis, Graft vs Host disease (GVHD), IgG4 related disease

In 2012, an alternative set of criteria were published and provisionally adopted by the American College of Rheumatology (ACR) for classification of PSS. These classification criteria use objective measures only, arguably leaving less potential for misdiagnosis, which is essential when considering advanced therapies such as biological agents [80].

**Provisional ACR Classification Criteria (2012)**

The classification of PSS will be met in patients demonstrating signs and symptoms of Sjögren's Syndrome and 2 out of 3 of the following objective features:

I. Positive serum anti-Ro or anti-La or positive rheumatoid factor and antinuclear antibody (ANA) titre of >1:320
II. Labial salivary gland biopsy exhibiting focal lymphocytic sialadenitis with focus score of >1 focus/4mm2
III. Keratoconjunctivitis sicca with ocular staining score $\geq$ 3

Exclusion criteria: History of head and neck radiation, Hepatitis C infection, Acquired immunodeficiency syndrome, Sarcoidosis, Amyloidosis, Graft vs host disease, IgG4 related disease.

Exclusion criteria for the ACR provisional criteria are the same as for the AECG criteria with the additional exclusion of IgG4 related disease. The ACR and AECG classification criteria yield concordant results in the majority of cases and gene expression profiling suggests that patients meeting either set of criteria are more similar to other SS participants than to healthy controls [84]. The development of consensus criteria by the ACR-European League Against Rheumatism (EULAR) working group to bring together the two criteria is currently in progress.

Criteria are never fixed in perpetuity and as new technologies such as ultrasound scanning (USS) become more widely used or new data becomes available [85] further revision is likely.

For example, one of the differences between the various criteria is whether to score a focus score of $\geq 1$ or $> 1$ as positive. Recent data suggests that the former is more closely linked with the clinical phenotype of PSS [86]. Improvements in diagnostic acumen may require a greater understanding of the pathogenic mechanisms underlying the disease. Agreed classification criteria are essential in clinical research so that there is confidence that participants in a study have the specified condition.

## Useful Investigations for the Diagnosis and Assessment of PSS

All patients with suspected PSS should undergo several basic investigations, including full blood count, urea and electrolytes, liver and thyroid function tests, creatinine kinase, inflammatory markers (e.g., erythrocyte sedimentation rate (ESR), C-reactive protein (CRP)), immunoglobulins and serum electrophoresis, complement levels, and autoantibody screen (including ANA, dsDNA, rheumatoid factor (RF) and anti-Ro (SSA) and anti-La (SSB)). Urine should be sampled for dipstick analysis, and a baseline chest x-ray should be requested (if not done in the last 6 months) [87]. Oral and ocular exocrine function should be assessed with Schirmer's I test and unstimulated whole saliva flow measurement.

There is increasing evidence that USS of the salivary glands is both sensitive and specific (82% and 73% respectively in a recent study by Takegi et al.) for detecting glandular structural changes [88-90]. USS has the benefits of being non-invasive, and can easily be repeated for longitudinal follow-up. It is, however, user-dependent, and therefore should only be performed by an experienced sonographer [88]. Minor salivary gland biopsy should be offered to all patients with suspected PSS as part of the diagnostic work-up. The sample is assessed for focal lymphocytic sialadenitis (the presence of a dense aggregate of 50 or more lymphocytes, generally in periductal or perivascular sites, is termed a "focus"). The histology sample is given a Focus Score (FS) according to the number of "focus" present within an examination field of $4mm^2$ [86]. Initial studies suggest that FS is associated with disease activity and a positive serum anti-Ro. Although specificity and positive predictive value is high, sensitivity is variable [91]. As such, the findings of minor labial salivary gland biopsy should be considered in the context of clinical findings as per the AECG criteria [92]. The detection of germinal centre-like structures by light microscopy in diagnostic salivary gland biopsies has been proposed as a highly predictive and easily obtainable marker of risk of developing non-Hodgkin lymphoma. Salivary gland biopsies may therefore allow for risk and therapeutic stratification (such as the use of B-cell directed therapy) [93]. Salivary gland function may be further assessed by glandular salivary collection and sialochemistry, MRI salivary glands and scintigraphy where indicated.

Ocular damage may be assessed by Lissamine green test, Rose Bengal staining or fluorescein staining. Referral to an ophthalmologist for further assessment may prompt further investigations such as tear film break up time, tear function index, impression cytology, tear osmolality and calculation of the ocular surface disease index.

If the diagnosis remains unclear or if an alternative diagnosis is suspected, physicians may also consider screening for Hepatitis A, B and C, Epstein Barr virus (EBV), Human immunodeficiency virus (HIV), and test for serum angiotensin converting enzyme (sACE), cryoglobulins and HbA1c.

## Differential Diagnosis of PSS

There are a number of conditions that are associated with sicca symptoms and/or salivary gland swelling. These include infective (HIV, Hepatitis A, B or C, Human T-cell lymphotropic virus 1 (HTLV-1), mumps, EBV, Cytomegalovirus (CMV), tuberculosis (TB)), inflammatory/immune-mediated (sarcoidosis, amyloidosis, IgG4-related disease), malignancy (lymphoma or other malignancy), iatrogenic (Graft versus host disease (GVHD), head and neck irradiation, medications), endocrine/metabolic (diabetes, acromegaly, alcohol excess, cirrhosis, lipoproteinaemia, bulimia, anorexia nervosa, endurance athletes, chronic pancreatitis) and miscellaneous (fibromyalgia, chronic fatigue syndrome, sialolithiasis, sialoadenitis) conditions [94].

Dry mouth is a common oral symptom and the majority of individuals with this complaint do not have a diagnosis of Sjögren's syndrome. The differential diagnosis of xerostomia can be classified according to the presence or absence of salivary gland disease with glandular hypofunction. Xerostomia can result from the adverse effects of drugs and diseases (See table 1.1). Although functioning acinar tissue in the salivary glands reduces with increasing age, it does not result in clinically significant gland hypofunction as the glands have a large secretory reserve [95].

**Table 1.1. Causes of Xerostomia**

| | |
|---|---|
| Iatrogenic | Drugs Anti-cholinergics (e.g., psychotropics including antidepressants, anxiolytics and anti-psychotics); muscarinic antagonists (e.g., tamsolusin hydrochloride; ipratropium hydrochloride); anti-histamines, opiates; anti-hypertensives (e.g., beta blockers; ACE inhibitors); proton pump inhibitors (e.g., omeprazole)<br>Head & neck radiotherapy<br>Graft versus host disease (which produces an analogous condition to Sjögren's syndrome) |
| "Physiological" | Dehydration (e.g., poorly controlled diabetes)<br>Acute anxiety<br>Mouth breathing |
| Other medical conditions | Renal failure<br>Sarcoidosis<br>Central lesions (rare)<br>Salivary gland aplasia and ductal atresia which may be related to FGF10 missense mutations [96](rare) |
| Infections | HIV-associated salivary gland disease (DILS)<br>Hepatitis C |
| Idiopathic | "SOX" (Sialoadenitis, Osteoarthritis, Xerostomia)<br>"Sicca syndrome" (dryness where there is no known obvious case for the salivary gland hypofunction) |

Oral dysaesthesia can result in the symptom of xerostomia with no objective reduction in salivary flow rate. Classically patients complain of abnormal taste and oral burning sensations, in addition to oral dryness. This is commonly associated with anxiety states and occasionally, clinical depression. Symptoms may co-exist with low back pain, fibromyalgia and irritable bowel syndrome [97]. A new clinical entity called 'Sialadenitis, Osteoarthritis, and Xerostomia (SOX)' has been described comprising histological evidence of non-specific sialadenitis, generalised nodular osteoarthritis and xerostomia [98]. However, given the frequency of the individual clinical features, the association may be due to clustering.

## Disease Assessment

In the absence of specific clinical or biological disease activity markers, a number of assessment tools specific to PSS have been developed in recent years. This has met the demand for a standardised and validated method of assessing patients in clinical trials and has become of increasing importance with the development of biologic therapies. The assessment tools may also be transferred to routine clinical practice, as a method of assessing the clinical course overtime and auditing outcomes.

## Ocular Assessment

Ocular assessment should ideally be performed by an ophthalmologist with the appropriate specialist equipment, skills and knowledge to perform a full assessment of ocular involvement, especially if the symptoms are severe. The Dry Eye Severity Grading Scheme is the most commonly used assessment tool, and takes into account discomfort (severity and frequency), visual symptoms, conjunctival injection, conjunctival staining, corneal staining, corneal/ tear signs (such as filamentary keratitis, mucus clumping, increased tear debris and ulceration), lid and MG involvement, tear break-up time and Schirmer's I score [6].

The Sicca Symptoms Inventory (SSI), EULAR Sicca Score (ESS) and ESSPRI (EULAR Sjögren's Syndrome Patient Reported Index) provide assessment of patient reported ocular and oral dryness using visual analogue scores. SSI assesses 42 aspects of sicca symptoms, relating to severity over the preceeding two weeks. Short and long versions of the form are available to provide a 'snap shot' of the patient's perspective of sicca symptoms [99]. Schirmer's tear tests, performed with or without topical local anaesthesia, can provide objective measurements of lacrimal gland function at bedside by non-ophthalmology clinicians or trained health care assistants.

Detailed discussion of the clinical tests utilised by specialist ophthalmologists in the assessment of PSS related dry eye is beyond the scope of this chapter. These tests include ocular surface vital staining (fluorescein, Lissamine green), tear film break up time (TFBUT), tear film osmolarity and impression cytology. Other objective assessment tools for quantifying disease include tear film proteomic analyses and ocular surface in vivo confocal microscopy, but are largely being used only in research settings.

## Oral Assessment

Xerostomia may be quantified by either stimulated or unstimulated salivary flow rates. This is a crude measure of salivary gland function, however it is easy to perform in clinical practice and appears sensitive to change, according to disease activity [100].

A history of salivary gland swelling should be elicited, the salivary gland areas should be examined and the findings documented. Hard or unilateral parotid gland enlargement should prompt further investigations with urgent salivary gland ultrasound or MRI and referral for biopsy to exclude a tumour. It is noteworthy that bilateral enlargement doesn't automatically exclude a malignant aetiology, warthin's tumour can occur bilaterally [101]. In addition, associated VII nerve motor weakness or palsy can complicate swelling of the lower pole of the parotid glands. Acute, unilateral parotitis when accompanied by fever, erythema and tenderness may be caused by infection, or obstruction. Intraoral milking of the salivary glands may yield thick mucoid saliva, infection is suggested by the presence of blood or pus. An important symptom which suggests obstructive aetiology is pain associated with eating. This may be due to intra-glandular ductal stenosis or malignant infiltration.

Oral and dental health and hygiene should be assessed regularly in conjunction with oral medicine specialists and dentists.

## Assessment of Extra-Glandular Disease

A structured approach to assessment of systemic involvement in PSS is essential. Differentiating between active disease activity and irreversible organ damage can be challenging. A number of tools have been developed and validated over recent years to provide enable structured assessment of systemic disease activities and end-organ damage.

## Systemic Disease Activity

EULAR has developed the EULAR Sjögren's Syndrome Disease Activity Index (ESSDAI) through international collaboration of an expert panel. The index measures the degree of disease activity in patients with systemic involvement. It covers a number of domains, including constitutional, lymphadenopathy, glandular, articular, cutaneous, pulmonary, renal, muscular, peripheral nervous system (PNS), CNS, haematological and biological. Each domain is scored if the condition is 'new' or 'worsening' in order to prevent repeatedly scoring damage, thus allowing comparison of scores between two time-points. ESSDAI demonstrates high content validity, reliability and sensitivity to change, allowing for comparison of results pre- and post-treatment, and between clinical trials [102, 103].

**Table 1.2. Adapted from Sjögren's Syndrome Management, Ng WF, Vissink A, Theander T, and Figueiredo F. Oxford Journals of Rheumatology (87)**

| Suggested structured assessment of systemic disease activity of pSS | | | |
|---|---|---|---|
| Organ systems | Symptoms | Signs | Clinical tests (if indicated) |
| Constitutional & lymphatic | Fatigue, fever, night sweat, weight loss (unintentional) | Fever, lymphadenopathy, splenomegaly | "Malignancy screen" with appropriate imaging and blood tests |
| Glandular | Glandular pain and swelling | Glandular tenderness and/or enlargement | Salivary gland USS/MRI |
| Articular | Arthralgia, early morning stiffness | Synovitis | X-ray, musculoskeletal USS |
| Cutaneous | Rash, pain, itch, skin ulceration or necrosis, cold extremities ± colour changes | Dry skin, rash (e.g., erythema multiforme, cutaneous vasculitis, urticaria, purpura, subacute cutaneous lupus), ulcer, Raynaud's phenomenon | Skin biopsy, full autoimmune screen (if not already done recently), cryoglobulin measurement, nailfold capillaroscopy |
| Pulmonary | Husky voice, breathlessness, persistent non-productive dry cough, chest pain | Pleural rub, crepitations, reduced breath sound, percussion dullness. | Chest radiograph, pulmonary function tests, HRCT chest |
| Renal | Muscle weakness, bone pain, fatigue, renal colic | (Inappropriately) Alkaline urine, hypercalciuria, urinary stone, proteinuria, haematuria | Electrolytes, serum chlorides, serum and urinary calcium & pH, renal USS |
| Muscular | Myalgia, weakness | Weakness | Serum CK, EMG, MRI muscles, muscle biopsy |

**Table 1.2. (Continued)**

| Suggested structured assessment of systemic disease activity of pSS | | | |
|---|---|---|---|
| Organ systems | Symptoms | Signs | Clinical tests (if indicated) |
| Peripheral nervous system | Paraesthesia, sensory deficit, weakness, ataxia, multiple sclerosis-like syndrome | Sensory changes, motor deficit, ataxia, mononeuritis multiplex | Neurophysiology, nerve biopsy, cyroglobulin measurement, ?Skin biopsy |
| Central nervous system | Multiple sclerosis-like syndrome, seizures, cognitive impairment, headache | Optic neuritis, transverse myelitis, cranial neuropathy, meningism | MRI/CT of brain/spinal cord, CSF examination ; fundoscopy |
| Haematological and biological | Fatigue, easy bruising | Anaemia, bruises | Full blood count, serum and urine Immunoglobulins levels and electrophoresis, Coombe's test, bone marrow examination |

Other systemic disease assessment tools have also been developed. Sjögren's Syndrome Disease Activity Index (SSDAI) is based on a large cohort of Italian patients with PSS. It has been shown to have good sensitivity and specificity (84·5% and 87·6% respectively) for differentiating the level of disease activity, and takes subjective measures (e.g., fatigue) into account. Its main weakness is that it also relies on the results of investigations which are invasive and/or cannot be repeated regularly (for example, CT thorax, electromyography (EMG), renal biopsy). Content validity may be affected as this study was performed in one country only [100, 104]. Similarly to SSDAI, Sjögren's Systemic Clinical Activity Index (SCAI) is based on a national study within a limited geographical area. The domain definitions are based on 'intention-to-treat', which reflect clinically relevant changes in disease activity. It also includes subjective domains including fatigue. The main criticism of this score is that the 'arthritis' domain correlates with osteoarthritis, and therefore may result in over-estimation of disease activity [105]. The use of SSDAI and SCAI are likely to be supplanted by the development of ESSDAI.

## End Organ Damage

### *Sjögren's Syndrome Disease Damage Index (SSDDI)*

The aim of SSDDI is to assess the accumulated, permanent morbidity due the disease and side- effects of treatment. It provides a global score of disease damage, giving weight to damage that is likely to result in more severe outcomes (brain, renal, malignancy). It demonstrates high construct validity by clearly defining damage as opposed to activity [100, 104].

### *Sjögren's Syndrome Damage Index (SSDI)*

SSDI assesses three domains: ocular, oral and systemic damage. It also provides a global damage score. The tool is not limited to implementation by specialists, and can be performed in any clinical setting without the use of equipment e.g., slit lamps. However, item response largely depends on clinician experience which in turn is likely to affect inter-rater reliability. It also fails to give weight to the more significant aspects of disease damage. It does differentiate between damage secondary to PSS or secondary to other co-morbidities [100, 106].

## Patient Reported Outcomes

The EULAR Sjögren's Syndrome Patient Reported Index (ESSPRI) provides an easy-to-use assessment of patient's symptom severity. It encompasses sicca symptoms, fatigue and health-related quality of life assessment using Likert's scales. It was constructed using a large multinational cohort, with high content validity. It has been shown to be a sensitive measure of change in disease activity after therapeutic intervention [103].

The Profile of Fatigue and Discomfort (PROFAD) measures somatic fatigue, mental fatigue, arthralgia and vascular dysfunction. It was designed to specifically measure fatigue of PSS, and is an important tool to assess what is often the most disabling symptom of PSS.

There are a number of other tools that may be considered for assessing patient quality of life, functional capacity and patient perspective of symptoms, including Epworth Sleepiness Scale, Orthostatic Symptoms Scale, EQ-5D, SF-36, and Hospital Anxiety and Depression Scale.

## Management

*To date, there are no agreed evidence-based guidelines on the management of PSS. The recommendations below are based on best available evidence. The* management strategy for PSS can be categorised into preventative, replacement or stimulatory interventions. The decision to treat is based on a combination of physician experience, expert consensus and reported studies.

### *Ocular*

Patients should be counselled on simple preventative measures such as avoiding dry environments (wind, air conditioning, central heating), good eye care, regular optician review, avoiding irritants (dust, cigarette smoke, contact lenses), and avoiding activities that exacerbate symptoms (prolonged reading or computer use) [107].

A number of drugs are recognised to exacerbate dry eye symptoms and should be avoided if possible. This list includes (but is not exhaustive) diuretics, beta-blockers, antihistamines and tricyclic antidepressants.

Conditions that exacerbate sicca symptoms, such as lagophthalmos, ectropion, and meibomian gland disease should be referred for prompt ophthalmology review.

Replacement of tear volume has been shown to palliate dry eye symptoms [108] and may also improve ocular surface disease (keratoconjunctivitis sicca) [109]. Tear substitutes act by reducing tear osmolality and lubricating the ocular surface. A recent systematic review of treatment for PSS [110] recommended frequent use of preservative-free tear substitutes during the day, while reserving lubricating ointments for nocturnal use. There are a range of either aqueous or lipid based preparations available. Efficacy and tolerance of the different preparations varies between patients and should be tailored to the individual.

Patients with severe refractory ocular dryness should be under the care of an ophthalmologist. Mucolytics may be considered for patients presenting with 'sticky eyes'. Topical glucocorticoids or NSAIDS may be prescribed for ocular inflammation, although the duration of use should be limited to 'pulsed' therapy due to the risk of adverse effects (raised intra-ocular pressure, cataracts). Controlled trials support the use of topical immuno-modulatory cyclosporine for moderate to severe dry eye disease. It has been shown to reduce the expression of pro-apoptotic markers within the conjunctival epithelium and improve objective and subjective measures of dry eye disease.

Emulsions, containing both aqueous and lipid components are recommended for use alongside water-insoluble ciclosporin drops [108]. Parasympathetic sialagogues pilocarpine or cevimaline have been shown to improve xerophthalmia as well as xerostomia (see below).

Punctal occlusion preserves the tear film by retarding tear reabsorption. It should be considered for severe keratoconjunctivitis sicca. Complications of punctual plugging include infection and extrusion or migration of plugs into the canaliculi. Permanent occlusion by surgical or cauterisation methods may also be considered [107].

MG deficiency is a common feature of PSS. Dysfunction of the gland results in loss of the lipid layer overlying the tear film, resulting in reduced tear break up time, increased risk of infection and inflammation, and punctate keratopathy. Patients may complain of stinging, burning and chronic inflammation of the eyelids. Treatment consists of maintaining lid hygiene: warm compresses, lid massage and lid scrubs. A short course of antibiotic/steroid drops may be beneficial in reducing inflammation [111]. Prophylactic chloramphenicol drops at night may be considered for recurrent conjunctivitis or blepharitis [94].

### *Oral*

Patients should be educated on the importance of robust oral and dental hygiene and regular dental review. Patients should avoid exacerbators of dry mouth if possible, these include mouth breathing, dry and spicy foods, alcohol and caffeine. They should also avoid exacerbating environment's, such as central heating, air conditioning, wind, dust, and cigarette smoke.

Other medical conditions that cause xerostomia, for example endocrine, metabolic or viral infections should be treated appropriately. Avoidance, reduction or substitution of xerostomising drugs such as anticholinergics, antihistamines, antihypertensives and neuroleptics is essential.

Saliva substitutes are thought to have limited effect on symptoms of dry mouth. They require repeated application due to swallowing, and therefore are generally reserved for moderate to severe symptoms. They act by lubricating the mouth, however they do not have the protective benefits of natural saliva. There are a number of preparations available in gel, oil, lozenge or spray form. Some of the preparations contain fluorides and re-mineralising solution, which is thought to confer some dental protection. Patients are encouraged to take regular sips of water and use sugar-free chewing gum or lozenges to stimulate the salivary glands [107].

Muscarinic agonists (pilocarpine, cevimaline) can significantly improve salivary secretion and relieve the symptoms of both xerostomia and xerophthalmia in patients with residual glandular function. However, their benefits must be weighed against possible side effects, including flushing, headache, nausea, diarrhoea and urinary frequency. The medication takes up to six weeks to reach its full effect. It should be avoided in patients with history of ischaemic heart disease and uncontrolled asthma [94].

Fungal infections can be treated with topical or systemic antifungals and soaking dentures overnight in chlorhexidine. Angular chelitis should be treated with topical combined antifungal/steroid cream or ointment.

### *Systemic (Extra-Glandular)*

#### Constitutional

Symptoms of anorexia, weight loss, fevers, night sweats and fatigue are frequent and may profoundly limit patient activity. If symptoms are severe, lymphoma should be excluded. There is some evidence to suggest that hydroxychloroquine or a short course of corticosteroids may alleviate symptoms, by lowering the levels of circulating immunoglobulins [94].

#### Articular & Muscular

Arthralgia is common although inflammatory arthritis is present in only 20% of patients. PSS patients tend to have a relapsing-remitting course as opposed to the progressive inflammation seen in RA. Early morning stiffness is a less prominent symptom in these patients. Treatment is with analgesia, short courses of oral corticosteroids where indicated, and hydroxychloroquine. PSS tend to be less responsive to other disease modifying agents [94].

Myalgia alone can be treated with NSAIDs or hydroxychloroquine. For patients with myositis (raised CK, confirmed on EMG or muscle biopsy), treatment is with steroids, methotrexate or azathioprine. A differential diagnosis of polymyalgia rheumatica, inclusion body myositis, myopathy due to statins or steroids, and fibromyalgia should be considered [41, 94].

#### Respiratory

Treatment of respiratory manifestations depends on their severity and may require corticosteroids or immunosuppression with cyclophosphamide for patients with significant interstitial/bronchial disease or reduced pulmonary function.

## Neurological

Treatment of peripheral neuropathy depends on the underlying cause. Small-fibre (pure sensory) neuropathy can be treated with analgesics or pain modifying treatments (such as gabapentin, amitriptyline, pregabalin, carbamazepine), but patients should be warned of the risk of exacerbating sicca symptoms. Hydroxychloroquine may slow the progression of sensorimotor polyneuropathy. Mononeuritis multiplex is treated with corticosteroids and cyclophosphamide. Patients with symptoms of autonomic dysfunction should be advised to maintain adequate hydration, use of compression stockings and avoid standing from sitting or lying too quickly. The use of midodrine or fludrocortisone should be reserved for patients with objective abnormal autonomic tests and in conjunction with a specialist with expertise in the treatment of autonomic dysfunction. Central nervous system manifestations are extremely rare and should be treated with corticosteroids and cyclophosphamide. Refractory cases may be treated with rituximab, plasmapheresis and intravenous immunoglobulin, particularly if related to a systemic vasculitis or cryoglobuliaemia [40].

## Cutaneous

Pruritus and dry skin should be managed symptomatically with topical emollients and antihistamines. Patients with photosensitivity should avoid prolonged sun exposure and use high factor sun block.

Mild cutaneous vasculitis can be managed with elevation of the legs, avoidance of prolonged standing and simple analgesia [112]. Dapsone or colchicine can be used for mild recurrent or persistent disease, whereas systemic corticosteroids or other immunosuppression (azathioprine, methotrexate or cyclophosphamide) may be required for more severe disease. If the vasculitis is systemic or resistant to these therapies, plasmapheresis, intravenous immunoglobulin or rituximab may be considered, particularly for those with cryoglobulinaemia [107].

Hydroxychloroquine and compression stockings may help alleviate symptoms of hypergammaglobulinaemia-associated purpura.

Precipitants such as smoking and beta blockers should be avoided in patients with Raynaud's phenomenon. Pharmacological treatments include calcium channel blockers, ACE-inhibitors and in severe cases intravenous prostacycline. Nailfold capillaroscopy can be useful diagnostically to differentiate between primary and secondary Raynaud's [113].

### Genitourinary

Symptoms of chronic cystitis may respond to cimetidine or low dose steroids [94].

Electrolyte abnormalities associated with renal tubular acidosis usually resolve with treatment with alkalis such as sodium bicarbonate or potassium citrate [94]. Review of nephrotoxic drugs in these patients is essential [41]. Glomerulonephritis requires treatment with corticosteroids, cyclophosphamide or plasmapheresis [107].

Lubricating gels and pessaries are recommended for dyspareunia. For post-menopausal patients, local oestrogen preparations can also be prescribed. Cortisone preparations are not recommended. Co-existing candida infections of the vulva or vagina should be treated conventionally.

### Gastrointestinal

Gastro-oesophageal reflux can be treated with proton pump inhibitors and eradication therapy for those with Helicobacter Pylori infections. Ursodeoxycholic acid is a useful treatment for co-existing PBC. Corticosteroids or azathioprine may be useful in patients with autoimmune hepatitis and persistently elevated liver function tests [40, 41].

### Haematological

Haematologic manifestations are usually mild and do not usually require treatment. More severe cytopenias may require input of a haematologist and treatment with immunosuppression [107].

### Fatigue

Effective management of fatigue remains a considerable challenge. Hydroxychloroquine is often tried. Patients should be given advice on avoiding exacerbating factors such as disturbed sleep, stress and depression. Graded exercise regimes may be beneficial. Medical conditions (e.g., hypothyroidism, anaemia, vitamin deficiencies, coeliac disease, renal disease) that may exacerbate fatigue should also be sought and treated appropriately [94].

### Lymphoma

Patients at 'high risk' for the development of lymphoma should be educated about the signs and symptoms of lymphoma which should prompt them to seek medical attention. High-risk patients should be reviewed on a 6 monthly basis and undergo complete physical examination (specifically of the accessible nodal areas), full blood count, biochemistry panel, serum protein electrophoresis, serum and urine immunofixation, serum complement and cryoglobulins levels.

Investigation of lymphoma, regardless of type and stage should include MRI or CT neck, chest, abdomen and pelvis, full blood count, biochemistry, lactate dehydrogenase (LDH) level, serum protein electrophoresis, complement levels, paraproteins, β2m, IgM RF, immunoglobulins and cryoglobulins, bone marrow aspiration and biopsy and where appropriate, oesophageal-gastro-duodenal endoscopy with multiple biopsies and H. Pylori testing. Any pulmonary opacities should be biopsied for detection of bronchial MALT lymphoma [16].

Treatment is usually managed by the haematologist or oncologist, and is tailored to the patient based on symptoms, site, grade, stage, and extent of lymphoma [114].

**Table 1.3. Summary of lymphoma types**

| Type | Localised extra-nodal marginal zone lymphoma | Disseminated extra-nodal marginal zone lymphoma or nodal | High grade transformation of MALT or DLBCL |
|---|---|---|---|
| Localisation | Localised to salivary glands | Regional lymph nodes | Disseminated disease |
| Metastases | No BM infiltration | Bone marrow infiltration, multiple mucosal and nodal involvement in advanced stages | Distant lymph nodes or bone marrow. |
| Symptoms | No B Symptoms | B Symptoms | B Symptoms |
| Prognosis | 5 year survival 90%. 10% convert to high grade malignant lymphomas. | Extra-nodal: 3 year overall survival of 97%, 3 year disease free survival of 80%<br>Nodal: 3 year survival 80%, 3 year disease free 50% | 3 year overall survival 100%, 3 year disease free survival 100% |
| Treatment (also depends on disease activity) | Observation<br>Surgical resection +/- radiotherapy | Surgical resection +/- radiotherapy<br>Rituximab – Cyclophosphamide and prednisolone (CHOP) x 6-8 if severe symptoms | Rituximab and CHOP x 6-8 |

## PSS in Pregnancy

PSS patients with anti-Ro antibodies who are pregnant should be closely monitored with weekly or fortnightly obstetric ultrasound scanning and echocardiography between 12 and 30 weeks of gestation, as this is the most common time for AV block to develop [94]. Neonates should be delivered and cared for in a tertiary centre with cardiac pacing facilities available if required. There is some evidence to suggest that treating the mother with high dose dexamethasone or betamethasone in early pregnancy can prevent foetal development of complete heart block. The outcome of these pregnancies is generally good with neonatal screening and management in a specialist setting.

## Emerging Therapies

There has been limited success of the currently available treatments for PSS. One reason for this may be that exocrine function has already been exhausted (due to delayed presentation and/or diagnosis) and therefore stimulation of the glands or attempts to prevent further damage is futile. Another possible explanation is that understanding of the underlying pathophysiology is limited and therefore treatment has not been duly targeted.

Over recent years there has been improved understanding of genetic and molecular abnormalities involved in the pathophysiological process in PSS in particular and a number of biological pathways have been identified for targeted treatment.

## B-Cell Targeted Therapy

B-cell hyperactivity and dysregulation is associated with PSS. Hypogammaglobulinaemia and antibody positivity (SSA/ Anti-Ro and SSB/Anti-La) is a common feature. Salivary gland biopsy demonstrates replacement of IgA producing plasma cells with IgG-producing plasma cells, and B-cell lymphoma is strongly associated with PSS.

Rituximab is an established and effective treatment for B-cell lymphoma and other autoimmune conditions, including RA and SLE. There have been a number of trials assessing the efficacy of rituximab on PSS. The efficacy of rituximab is summarised in the table below based on published clinical data to date.

**Table 1.4. Summary of Evidence for Rituximab**

| *Symptom/Sign* | *Evidence* | *Comment* |
|---|---|---|
| *Sicca symptoms* | Conflicting | Rituximab more effective at improving sicca symptoms in early disease when there is residual glandular function. Good response to subjective measures, poor response to objective measures. |
| *Joint symptoms* | Significant improvement | |
| *Fatigue* | Significant improvement | Improvement in fatigue VAS, MFI and SF-36 |
| *Systemic features* | Significant improvement | Improvement has been demonstrated in cryoglobulinaemia, cutaneous vasculitis, polyarthritis, pulmonary involvement, renal involvement, thrombocytopenia and autoimmune pancreatitis. Less response in CNS/PNS/Myositis. |
| *Lymphoma* | Effective | Treatment success increased if rituximab used in combination with other chemotherapies. |
| *EULAR outcome tools* | Improvement | More improvement of ESSDAI that ESSPRI |

The incidence of rituximab-associated infusion reactions including hypersensitivity, cytokine release syndrome and serum-sickness symptoms appear to be more common among PSS patients than patients with non-autoimmune conditions [115, 116].

The cytokine B-cell activation factor (BAFF) regulates B-cell proliferation and differentiation. It has been shown to be elevated in the serum and salivary gland biopsies of PSS patients. The monoclonal antibody belimumab targets BAFF. There are a number of studies currently in progress assessing its efficacy in PSS patients.

## T-Cell Targeted Therapy

T-cells are the predominant cell found in the inflammatory tissue of salivary glands. They mediate gland damage both directly and indirectly via T-helper cytokines. Abatacept, a fusion protein targeting the interaction between

T-cell and antigen presenting cells has shown some encouraging results in a phase II clinical trial (published abstracts only).

## Cytokine-Targeted Therapy

Many different cytokines have been shown to be up-regulated in the salivary glands of PSS patients [117]. Their role has yet to be clearly defined. A number of trials have investigated the benefit of monoclonal antibodies to IL-6 (tocilizumab), IL-12, IL-17 and IL-23 in other autoimmune conditions, however there is no published data in PSS to date. A recent study using an IL-1 receptor antagonist (anakinra) for the treatment of PSS related fatigue did not show any significant benefit over placebo [118].

## Type I Interferon (IFN) Targeted Therapy

IFN-α activity is increased in the sera and salivary gland in PSS. It has been postulated that increased IFN-α activity upregulates BAFF, MHC, CD40 and Fas expression in salivary glands. At least two monoclonal antibodies targeting IFN-α have been developed and are under investigation for the treatment of SLE, however research into efficacy for PSS has yet to be carried out.

### *IFN-α2*

Research into the efficacy of INF-α2 has shown mixed results. Treatment rationale is based on the theory that PSS may be the result of recurrent viral infection, and that it may increase aquaporin expression. It is an established treatment for Hepatitis C-induced sialadenitis, for example. However, recent studies have in fact demonstrated IFN-α2 involvement in the pro-inflammatory cytokine pathway of PSS [119]. The treatment of PSS with IFN-α2 requires further research.

## TNF-α Targeted Therapies

TNF-α blockade with infliximab and etanercept has shown disappointing results, one reason for this may be the compensatory up-regulation of other cytokines involved in the inflammatory process [120].

## Conclusion

PSS is a chronic autoimmune disease, characterised by lymphocytic infiltration of exocrine glands causing progressive destruction, with diverse extra-glandular features. It is a diagnostic challenge due to the broad differential diagnosis and lack of a unique diagnostic test. Dryness, fatigue and musculoskeletal pain are the hallmarks of this disease, as well as a spectrum of systemic manifestations. A number of assessment tools have been validated for monitoring both disease activity and disease damage such as ESSPRI and ESSDAI. The best practice approach to management involves utilising a multidisciplinary team including oral medicine, ophthalmology and rheumatology with other medical and allied health professional involvement depending on the presentation. Therapeutic options for sicca symptoms are limited to preventative measures and replacement therapies. The use of muscarinic agonists is limited due to their adverse effects, and traditional disease modifying agents have failed to demonstrate convincing efficacy. There are promising results for immuno-modulatory therapy from emerging studies.

## References

[1] H Sjögren. Zur kenntnis der keratoconjunctivitis sicca. *Acta Ophthalmol.* 1933; 11 (suppl II):1-151.

[2] J. Mikulicz. Uber eine eigenartige symmetrische Erkrankung der Tranen- und Mundspeicheldrusen. *Beitr. Chir. Fortschr. Stuttgart.* 1892;In: Billroth GT, ed.:610-30.

[3] WF Ng, Bowman SJ, B Griffiths, group UKPSSR study. United Kingdom Primary Sjogren's Syndrome Registry--a united effort to tackle an orphan rheumatic disease. *Rheumatology* (Oxford). 2011;Jan; 50(1):32-9.

[4] M Ramos-Casals, P Brito-Zerón, Solans R, MT Camps, A Casanovas, B Sopeña, et al. Systemic involvement in primary Sjogren's syndrome evaluated by the EULAR-SS disease activity index: analysis of 921 Spanish patients (GEAS-SS Registry). *Rheumatology* (Oxford). 2013;Oct 25.

[5] M Ramos-Casals, R Solans, J Rosas, MT Camps, A Gil, J Del Pino-Montes, et al. Primary Sjögren syndrome in Spain: clinical and

immunologic expression in 1010 patients. *Medicine* (Baltimore) 2008;87:210-9.

[6] The definition and classification of dry eye disease: report of the Definition and Classification Subcommittee of the International Dry Eye WorkShop (2007). *Ocular Surface.* 2007;5(2):75-93.

[7] ME Stern, RW Beuerman, al Fox RI et. The Pathology of Dry Eye: The Interaction Between the Ocular Surface and Lacrimal Glands. *Cornea.* 1998;17(6):584.

[8] C Baudouin. The pathology of dry eye. *Surv. Ophthalmol.* 2001;Mar;45(Suppl 2):S211-20.

[9] KK Nichols, GN Foulks, al Bron AJ et. The International Workshop on Meibomian Gland Dysfunction: Executive Summary. *Invest. Ophthalmol. Vis. Sci.* 2011;52(4):1922-9.

[10] IS Tuisku, YT Konttinen, LM Konttinen, TM Tervo. Alterations in corneal sensitivity and nerve morphology in patients with primary Sjögren's syndrome. *Exp. Eye Res.* 2008;86(6):879-85.

[11] H Liu, C Begley, al Chen M et. A Link between Tear Instability and Hyperosmolarity in Dry Eye. *Invest. Ophthalmol. Vis. Sci.* 2009; 50(8):3671-9.

[12] CS De Paiva, RM Corrales, al Villarreal AL et. Corticosteroid and doxycycline suppress MMP-9 and inflammatory cytokine expression, MAPK activation in the corneal epithelium in experimental dry eye. *Exp. Eye Res.* 2006;83(3):526-35.

[13] P Rosenthal, B Inna, D Jacobs. Corneal pain without stain: Is it real? *The Ocular Surface.* 2009;7(1):28-40.

[14] R Seror, H Bootsma, SJ Bowman, T Dörner, JE Gottenberg, X Mariette, et al. Outcome measures for primary Sjögren's syndrome. *J. Autoimmun.* 2012;Aug;39(1-2):97-102.

[15] J Pijpe, WW Kalk, H Bootsma, FK Spijkervet, CG Kallenberg, A. Vissink. Progression of salivary gland dysfunction in patients with Sjögren's syndrome. *Annals of the rheumatic diseases.* 2007; 66(1):107-12.

[16] R Solans-Laqué, A López-Hernandez, JA Bosch-Gil, A Palacios, M Campillo, M Vilardell-Tarres. Risk, Predictors, and Clinical Characteristics of Lymphoma Development in Primary Sjögren's Syndrome. *Seminars in Arthritis and Rheumatism.* 2011;41(3):415-23.

[17] AL Fauchais, B Ouattara, G Gondram, F Lalloue, D Petit, K Ly, et al. Articular manifestations in primary Sjogren's syndrome: clinical

significance and prognosis of 188 patients. *Rheumatology* (Oxford). 2010;49:1164-72.

[18] O Palm, T Garen, T Berge Enger, JL Jensen, MB Lund, TM Aaløkken, et al. Clinical pulmonary involvement in primary Sjogren's syndrome: prevalence, quality of life and mortality--a retrospective study based on registry data. *Rheumatology* (Oxford). 2013 Jan;52(1):173-9.

[19] V Yazisiz, G Arslan, IH Ozbudak, S Turker, F Erbasan, AB Avci, et al. Lung involvement in patients with primary Sjögren's syndrome: what are the predictors? *Rheumatol Int* 2010;Aug;30(10):1317-24.

[20] SM Yan, Y Zhao, XF Zeng, FC Zhang, Y Dong. Lung involvement of primary Sjögren's syndrome. [Article in Chinese]. *Zhonghua Jie He He Hu Xi Za Zhi.* 2008;31(7):513-6.

[21] R Egashira, T Kondo, T Hirai, N Kamochi, M Yakushiji, al Yamasaki F et. CT Findings of Thoracic Manifestations of Primary Sjögren Syndrome: Radiologic-Pathologic Correlation. *Radiographics.* 2013;33(7):1933-49.

[22] V Dalvi, EB Gonzalez, L Lovett. Lymphocytic interstitial pneumonitis (LIP) in Sjögren's syndrome: a case report and a review of the literature. *Clin Rheum.* 2007;26(8):1339-43.

[23] M Alkhayer, BG McCann, BD Harrison. Lymphocytic interstitial pneumonitis in association with Sjogren's syndrome. *Br J Dis Chest.* 1988; Jul;82(3):305-9.

[24] PP Pavlakis, H Alexopoulos, ML Kosmidis, I Mamali, HM Moutsopoulos, AG Tzioufas, et al. Peripheral neuropathies in Sjögren's syndrome: a critical update on clinical features and pathogenetic mechanisms. *J Autoimmun.* 2012 Aug;39(1-2):27-33.

[25] D Sène, M Jallouli, JP Lefaucheur, D Saadoun, N Costedoat-Chalumeau, T Maisonobe, et al. Peripheral neuropathies associated with primary Sjogren's syndrome: immunologic profiles of nonataxic sensory neuropathy and sensorimotor neuropathy. *Medicine* (Baltimore). 2011.;90(2):133-8.

[26] S Delalande, J de Seze, AL Fauchais, E Hachulla, T Stojkovic, D Ferriby, et al. Neurologic Manifestations in Primary Sjogren Syndrome: A Study of 82 Patients. *Medicine (Baltimore).* 2004;83(5):280-91.

[27] FZ Cai, S Lester, al. Lu T et. Mild autonomic dysfunction in primary Sjogren's syndrome: a controlled study. *Arthritis Res Ther.* 2008;10(2):R31.

[28] L Kovacs, D Paprika, al Takacs R et. Cardiovascular autonomic dysfunction in primary Sjogren's syndrome. *Rheumatology* (Oxford). 2004;43(1):95-9.

[29] T Mandl, O Hammar, E Theander, al et. Autonomic nervous dysfunction development in patients with primary Sjogren's syndrome: a follow-up study. *Rheumatology* (Oxford). 2010;49(6):1101-6.

[30] JL Newton, J Frith, D Powell, al et. Autonomic symptoms are common and are associated with overall symptom burden and disease activity in primary Sjogren's syndrome. *Ann. Rheum. Dis.* 2012;Dec;71(12):1973-9.

[31] M Ramos-Casals, JM Anaya, M García-Carrasco, J Rosas, A Bové, G Claver, et al. Cutaneous vasculitis in primary Sjögren syndrome. Classification and clinical significance of 52 patients. *Medicine* (Baltimore). 2004;83:96-106.

[32] BK Davidson, CA Kelly, 1999 Griffiths ID. Primary Sjögren's syndrome in the North East of England: a long-term follow-up study. *Rheumatology* (Oxford) 1999;Mar 83(3):245-53.

[33] M García-Carrasco, A Sisó, M Ramos-Casals, J Rosas, G de la Red, V Gil, et al. Raynaud's phenomenon in primary Sjögren's syndrome. Prevalence and clinical characteristics in a series of 320 patients. *J. Rheumatol*. 2002;Apr 29(4):726-30.

[34] J Walker, T Gordon, S Lester, S Downie-Doyle, D McEvoy, K Pile, et al. Increased severity of lower urinary tract symptoms and daytime somnolence in primary Sjögren's syndrome. *J. Rheumatol.* 2003;Nov 30(11):2406-12.

[35] m Tischler, D Caspi, Y Almog, R Segal, M Yaron. Increased incidence of urinary tract infection in patients with rheumatoid arthritis and secondary Sjogren’s syndrome. *Ann. Rheum. Dis.* 1992;51(2):604-6.

[36] AV Goules, IP Tatouli, HM Moutsopoulos, AG Tzioufas. Clinically significant renal involvement in primary Sjögren's syndrome: clinical presentation and outcome. *Arthritis Rheum.* 2013;Nov 65(11):2945-53.

[37] S Lehrer, E Bogursky, M Yemini, NG Kase, A Birkenfield. Gynaecologic manifestatons of Sjogren’s syndrome. *Am. J. Obstet. Gynecol.* 1994;170(3):835-7.

[38] LM Luft, SG Barr, LO Martin, EKL Chan, MJ Fritzler. Autoantibodies to tissue transglutaminase in Sjogren’s syndrome and related rheumatic diseases. *J. Rheumatol.* 2003;30(12):2613-9.

[39] C Selmi, PL Meroni, ME Gershwin. Primary biliary cirrhosis and Sjögren's syndrome: autoimmune epithelitis. *J. Autoimmun.* 2012; Aug;39(1-2):34-42.

[40] CP Mavragani, HM Moutsopoulos. Conventional Therapy of Sjögren's Syndrome. *Clinical Reviews in Allergy & Immunology*. 2007; 32:284-91.

[41] R Fox. Sjögren's syndrome. *The Lancet*. 2005;366(9482):321-31.

[42] PA Ostuni, G Gazzetto, F Chieco-Bianchi, B Riga, M Plebani, C Betterle, et al. Pancreatic exocrine involvement in primary Sjogren's syndrome. *Scand. J. Rheumatol.* 1996;25(1):47-51.

[43] JG Zhou, YF Qing, L Jiang, QB Yang, WF Luo. Clinical analysis of primary Sjögren's syndrome complicating anemia. *Clin. Rheumatol.* 2010;May;29(5):525-9.

[44] P Brito-Zerón, M Ramos-Casals, A Bove, J Sentis, J Font. Predicting adverse outcomes in primary Sjogren's syndrome: identification of prognostic factors. *Rheumatology* (Oxford). 2007;Aug 46(8):1359-62.

[45] C Baldini, P Pepe, L Quartuccio, R Priori, E Bartoloni, A Alunno, et al. Primary Sjogren's syndrome as a multi-organ disease: impact of the serological profile on the clinical presentation of the disease in a large cohort of Italian patients. *Rheumatology* (Oxford). 2013;Dec 24. [Epub ahead of print].

[46] EJ Borg, AP Risselada, JC Kelder. Relation of systemic autoantibodies to the number of extraglandular manifestations in primary Sjogren's syndrome : a retrospective analysis of 65 patients in the Netherlands. *Semin. Arth. Rheum.* 2011;40(6):547-51.

[47] ML Davies, EJ Taylor, C Gordon, SP Young, K Welsh, M Bunce, et al. Candidate T Cell Epitopes of the Human La/SSB Autoantigen. *Arthritis Rheum.* 2002;46:209-14.

[48] CP Mavragani, AG Tzioufas, 2000 Moutsopoulos HM. Sjögren's syndrome: autoantibodies to cellular antigens. Clinical and molecular aspects. *Int. Arch. Allergy Immunol.* 2000;Sep;123(1):46-57.

[49] M Rischmueller, S Lester, Z Chen, G Champion, R Van Den Berg, R Beer, et al. HLA class II phenotype controls diversification of the autoantibody response in primary Sjögren's syndrome (pSS). *Clin. Exp. Immunol.* 1998;111:365-71.

[50] Q Qin, H Wang, HZ Wang, YL Huang, H Li, WW Zhang, et al. Diagnostic accuracy of anti-alpha-fodrin antibodies for primary Sjögren's syndrome. *Mod. Rheumatol.* 2013.

[51] LJ Dawson, HE Allison, J Stanbury, D Fitzgerald, PM Smith. Putative anti-muscarinic antibodies cannot be detected in patients with primary Sjogren's syndrome using conventional immunological approaches. *Rheumatology* (Oxford). 2004 Dec;43(12):1488-95.

[52] T Sumida, H Tsuboi, M Iizuka, T Hirota, H Asashima, I Matsumoto. The role of M3 muscarinic acetylcholine receptor reactive T cells in Sjögren's syndrome: A critical review. *J. Autoimmun.*

[53] M Pertovaara, F Bootorabi, M Kuuslahti, A Pasternack, S Parkkila. Novel carbonic anhydrase autoantibodies and renal manifestations in patients with primary Sjogren's syndrome. *Rheumatology* (Oxford). 2011;Aug;50(8):1453-7.

[54] S Winer, I Astsaturov, R Cheung, H Tsui, A Song, R Gaedigk, et al. Primary Sjögren's syndrome and deficiency of ICA69. *Lancet.* 2002;360:1063-9.

[55] R Estiasari, T Matsushita, K Masaki, T Akiyama, T Yonekawa, N Isobe, et al. Comparison of clinical, immunological and neuroimaging features between anti-aquaporin-4 antibody-positive and antibody-negative Sjogren's syndrome patients with central nervous system manifestations. *Mult. Scler.* 2012;Jun;18(6):807-16.

[56] S Steinfeld, E Cogan, LS King, P Agre, R Kiss, C Delporte. Abnormal distribution of aquaporin-5 water channel protein in salivary glands from Sjögren’s syndrome patients. *Lab. Invest.* 2001;81:143-8.

[57] LJ Jara, C Navarro, P Brito-Zerón Mdel, M García-Carrasco, RO Escárcega, M. Ramos-Casals. Thyroid disease in Sjögren's syndrome. *Clin. Rheumatol*. 2007;Oct; 26(10):1601-6.

[58] J Coll, J Anglada, S Tomas, P Reth, A Goday, M Millan, et al. High prevalence of subclinical Sjogren’s syndrome features in patients with autoimmune thyroid disease. *J. Rheumatol.* 1997;24(9):1719-24.

[59] SJ Johnsen, JG Brun, LG Gøransson, MC Småstuen, TB Johannesen, K Haldorsen, et al. Risk of non-Hodgkin's lymphoma in primary Sjögren's syndrome: a population-based study. *Arthritis Care Res.* 2013; May;65(5):816-21.

[60] KL Hon, AK Leung. Neonatal Lupus Erythematosus. *Autoimmune Disease* 2012.

[61] SZ Hussein, LT Jacobsson, PG Lindquist, E Theander. Pregnancy and fetal outcome in women with primary Sjögren’s syndrome compared with women in the general population: a nested case control study. *Rheumatology* (Oxford). 2011;50(9):1612-7.

[62] S De Carolis, S Salvi, A Botta, S Garofalo, C Garufi, Ferrazzani, et al. The impact of primary Sjogren's syndrome on pregnancy outcome: Our series and review of the literature. *Autoimmunity Reviews.* 2014;13(2):103-7.

[63] D Lendrem, S Mitchell, P McMeekin, S Bowman, E Price, CT Pease, et al. Health-related utility values of patients with primary Sjogren's syndrome and its predictors. *Ann. Rheum. Dis.* 2013.
[64] B Segal, SJ Bowman, PC Fox, al et. Primary Sjogren's syndrome: health experiences and predictors of health quality among patients in the United States. *Health Qual Life Outcomes*. 2009;27(7):46.
[65] JM Meijer, PM Meiners, JJ Huddleston Slater, FK Spijkervet, CG Kallenberg, A Vissink, et al. Health-related quality of life, employment and disability in patients with Sjögren's syndrome. *Rheumatology* (Oxford, England). 2009;48(9):1077-82.
[66] B Strömbeck, C Ekdahl, R Manthorpe, al et. Health-related quality of life in primary Sjogren's syndrome, rheumatoid arthritis and fibromyalgia compared to normal population data using SF-36. *Scand. J. Rheumatol.* 2000;29:20-8.
[67] EK Tensing, SA Solovieva, T Tervahartiala, al et. Fatigue and health profile in sicca syndrome of Sjogren's and non-Sjogren's syndrome origin. *Clin. Exp. Rheumatol.* 2001;19:313-6.
[68] J Rostron, S Rogers, L Longman, al et. Health-related quality of life in patients with primary Sjogren's syndrome and xerostomia: a comparative study. *Gerodontology*. 2002;19:53-9.
[69] R Belenguer, M Ramos-Casals, P Brito-Zerón, al et. Influence of clinical and immunological parameters on the health-related quality of life in patients with primary Sjogren's syndrome. *Clin. Exp. Rheumatol.* 2005;23:351-6.
[70] J Champey, E Corruble, JE Gottenberg, al et. Quality of life and psychological status in patients with primary Sjogren's syndrome and sicca symptoms without autoimmune features. *Arthritis Rheum.* 2006;55:451-7.
[71] CM Stewart, KM Berg, S Cha, WH Reeves. Salivary dysfunction and quality of life in Sjogren's syndrome: a critical oral-systemic connection. *J. Am. Dent. Assoc.* 2008;139:291-9.
[72] P López-Jornet, F Camacho-Alonso. Quality of life in patients with Sjogren's syndrome and sicca complex. *J. Oral Rehabil.* 2008;35:875-81.
[73] R Baturone, M Soto, M Marquez, al et. Health-related quality of life in patients with primary Sjogren's syndrome: relationship with serum levels of proinflammatory cytokines. *Scand. J. Rheumatol*. 2009;2:1-4.
[74] N Sutcliffe, T Stoll, S Pyke, DA Isenberg. Functional disability and end organ damage in patients with systemic lupus erythematosus (SLE), SLE

and Sjögren's syndrome (SS), and primary SS. *J. Rheumatol.* 1998;25(1):63-8.

[75] SJ Bowman, DA Booth, RG Platts, Group UK Sjögren's Interest. Measurement of fatigue and discomfort in primary Sjogren's syndrome using a new questionnaire tool. *Rheumatology* (Oxford). 2004;43(Jun):758-64.

[76] CT Lwin, M Bishay, RG Platts, DA Booth, SJ Bowman. The assessment of fatigue in primary Sjögren's syndrome. *Scand. J. Rheumatol.* 2003;32(1):33-7.

[77] M Voulgarelis, AG Tzioufas, HM. Moutsopoulos. Mortality in Sjögren's syndrome. *Clin. Exp. Rheumatol.* 2008;26((5 Suppl 51)):S66-71.

[78] E Theander, R Manthorpe, LT Jacobsson. Mortality and causes of death in primary Sjögren's syndrome: a prospective cohort study. *Arthritis Rheum.* 2004;50:1262-9.

[79] SJ Bowman, Y St Pierre, N Sutcliffe, DA Isenberg, F Goldblatt, E Price, et al. Estimating indirect costs in primary Sjögren's syndrome. *The Journal of Rheumatology*. 2010;37:1010-5.

[80] SC Shiboski, CH Shiboski, L Criswell, A Baer, S Challacombe, H Lanfranchi, et al. American College of Rheumatology Classification Criteria for Sjögren's Syndrome: A Data-Driven, Expert Consensus Approach in the Sjögren's International Collaborative Clinical Alliance Cohort. *Arthritis Care & Research*. 2012;64(4):475-87.

[81] R Manthorpe, V Anderson, OA Jensen, P Oxholm, JU Prause, M Schiodt. Editorial comments to the four sets of criteria for Sjogren's syndrome. *Scand. J. Rheumatol.* 1986(suppl 61):31-5.

[82] C Vitali, S Bombardieri, HM Moutsopoulos, G Balestrieri, W Bencivelli, RM Bernstein, et al. Preliminary criteria for the classification of Sjögren's syndrome. Results of a prospective concerted action supported by the European Community. *Arthritis Rheum.* 1993 Mar;36(3):340-7.

[83] C Vitali, S Bombardieri, R Jonsson, HM Moutsopoulos, EL Alexander, SE Carsons, et al. Classification criteria for Sjögren's syndrome: a revised version of the European criteria proposed by the American-European Consensus Group. *Annals of the Rheumatic Diseases.* 2002;61:554-8.

[84] A Rasmussen, JA Ice, H Li, K Grundahl, JA Kelly, L Radfar, et al. Comparison of the American-European Consensus Group Sjogren's syndrome classification criteria to newly proposed American College of

Rheumatology criteria in a large, carefully characterised sicca cohort. *Ann. Rheum. Dis*. 2014;73(1):31-8.

[85] JP Whitcher, CH Shiboski, SC Shiboski, AM Heidenreich, K Kitagawa, S Zhang, et al. Sjögren's International Collaborative Clinical Alliance Research Groups. A simplified quantitative method for assessing keratoconjunctivits sicca from the Sjogren's Syndrome International Registry. *Am. J. Ophthalmol.* 2010;149:405-15.

[86] TE Daniels, D Cox, CH Shiboski, M Schiodt, A Wu, H Lanfranchi, et al. Associations between salivary gland histopathologic diagnoses and phenotypic features of Sjögren's syndrome (SS) among 1726 registry participants. *Arthritis Rheum.* 2011;63(7):2021-30.

[87] WF Ng, A Vissink, E Theander, F Figueiredo. 7.8.2 Sjogren's Syndrome Management. *Oxford textbook of Rheumatology*. 4th ed2013.

[88] RK Niemelä, R Takalo, E Pääkkö, I Suramo, M Päivänsalo, T Salo, et al. Ultrasonography of salivary glands in primary Sjögren's syndrome. A comparison with magnetic resonance imaging and magnetic resonance sialography of parotid glands. *Rheumatology* (Oxford). 2004;43(7): 875-9.

[89] S Ali, J Brown, R Ngu, T Daniels, J Greenspan, E Odell, et al. Correlation between ultrasound imaging of major salivary glands and histopathological findings of labial gland biopsy samples in Sjögren's syndrome. *The Lancet.* 2013;381(S1):19.

[90] Y Takagi, Y Kimura, H Nakamura, M Sasaki, K Eguchi, T Nakamura. Salivary gland ultrasonography: can it be an alternative to sialography as an imaging modality for Sjögren's syndrome? *Annals of the Rheumatic Diseases.* 2010;69:1321 - 4.

[91] D Guellec, D Cornec, S Jousse-Joulin, T Marhadour, P Marcorelles, JO Pers, et al. Diagnostic value of labial minor salivary gland biopsy for Sjögren's syndrome: a systematic review. *Autoimmunity Reviews.* 2013;12(3):416-20.

[92] P Morbini, A Manzo, R Caporali, O Epis, C Villa, C Tinelli, et al. Multilevel examination of minor salivary gland biopsy for Sjögren's syndrome significantly improved diagnostic performance of AECG classification criteria. *Arthritis Research & Therapy* 2005;7(2):R343-R8.

[93] E Theander, L Vasaitis, E Baecklund, G Nordmark, G Warfvinge, R Liedholm, et al. Lymphoid organisation in labial salivary gland biopsies is a possible predictor for the development of malignant lymphoma in primary Sjögren's syndrome. *Annals of the Rheumatic Diseases.* 2011;70: 1363-8.

[94] P.J Venables. Management of Patients Presenting with Sjögren's Syndrome. Best Practice & Research. *Clinical Rheumatology.* 2006;20(4):791-807.

[95] D Fischer, JA Ship. Effect of age on variability of parotid salivary gland flow rates over time. *Age Ageing.* 1999 28(6):557-61.

[96] M Entesarian, J Dahlqvist, V Shashi, al et. FGF10 missense mutations in aplasia of lacrimal and salivary glands. *Eur. J. Hum. Genet.* 2007;15:379-82.

[97] MD Mignogna, A Pollio, G Fortuna, al et. Unexplained somatic comorbidities in patients with burning mouth syndrome: a controlled clinical study. *Journal of Orofacial Pain* 2011;25(2):131-40.

[98] DG Kassimos, PJ Shirlaw, EHS Choy, al et. Chronic Sialadenitis in patients with nodal osteoarthritis. *Br. J. Rheumatol.* 1997;36:1312-217.

[99] SJ Bowman, DA Booth, RG Platts, A Field, J Rostron, Group the UK Sjögren's Interest. Validation of the Sicca Symptoms Inventory for clinical studies of Sjögren's syndrome. *Journal of Rheumatology.* 2003;30(6):1259-66.

[100] Campar A, Isenberg DA. Primary Sjögren's syndrome activity and damage indices comparison. *European Journal of Clinical Investigation.* 2010;40:636-44.

[101] HM Chedid, A Rapoport, KF Aikawa, S Menezes Ados, OA Curioni. Warthin's tumor of the parotid gland: study of 70 cases. *Rev. Col. Bras. Cir.* 2011;38(2):90-4.

[102] R Seror, P Ravaud, SJ Bowman, G Baron, A Tzioufas, E Theander, et al. EULAR Sjogren's syndrome disease activity index: development of a consensus systemic disease activity index for primary Sjogren's syndrome. *Annals of the Rheumatic Diseases.* 2010;69(6):1103-9.

[103] PM Meiners, S Arends, E Brouwer, FK Spijkervet, A Vissink, H Bootsma. Responsiveness of disease activity indices ESSPRI and ESSDAI in patients with primary Sjögren's syndrome treated with rituximab. *Annals of the Rheumatic Diseases.* 2012;71(8):1297-302.

[104] C Vitali, G Palombi, C Baldini, M Benucci, S Bombardieri, M Covelli, et al. Sjögren's Syndrome Disease Damage Index and Disease Activity Index Scoring Systems for the Assessment of Disease Damage and Disease Activity in Sjögren's Syndrome, Derived From an Analysis of a Cohort of Italian Patients. *Arthritis & Rheumatism.* 2007;56(7):2223-31.

[105] SJ Bowman, N Sutcliffe, DA Isenberg, F Goldblatt, M Adler, E Price. Sjögren's Systemic Clinical Activity Index (SCAI)-a systemic disease

activity measure for use in clinical trials in primary Sjögren's syndrome. *Rheumatology* (Oxford). 2007;46:1845-51.

[106] RJ Barry, N Sutcliffe, DA Isenberg, E Price, F Goldblatt, M Adler, et al. The Sjögren's Syndrome Damage Index-a damage index for use in clinical trials and observational studies in primary Sjögren's syndrome. *Rheumatology* (Oxford). 2008;47:1193-8.

[107] A Thanou-Stavraki, JA James. Primary Sjogren's Syndrome: Current and Prospective Therapies. *Seminars in Arthritis and Rheumatism.* 2008;37(5):273-92.

[108] G.N. Foulks. The evolving treatment of dry eye. *Ophthalmology Clinics of North America.* 2003;16:29-35.

[109] P Marsh, SC Pflugfelder. Topical nonpreserved methylprednisolone therapy for keratoconjunctivitis sicca in Sjögren syndrome. *Ophthalmology Clinics of North America.* 1999;106(4):811-6.

[110] M Ramos-Casals, AG Tzioufas, JH Stone, A Siso, X Bosch. Treatment of primary Sjögren's syndrome: a systematic review. *The Journal of the American Medical Association* 2010;304(4):452-60.

[111] PJ Driver, MA Lemp. Meibomian gland dysfunction. *Survey of Ophthalmology.* 1996;40(5):343-67.

[112] KR Chen, JA Carlson. Clinical Approach to Cutaneous Vasculitis. *American Journal of Clinical Dermatology.* 2008;9(2):71-92.

[113] S Pavlov-Dolijanovic, NS Damjanov, RM Stojanovic, NZ Vujasinovic Stupar, DM Stanisavljevic. Scleroderma pattern of nailfold capillary changes as predictive value for the development of a connective tissue disease: a follow-up study of 3,029 patients with primary Raynaud's phenomenon. *Rheumatol Int.* 2012;32(10):3039-45.

[114] JG Routsias, JD Goules, G Charalampakis, S Tzima, A Papageorgiou, M Voulgarelis. Malignant lymphoma in primary Sjögren's syndrome: An update on the pathogenesis and treatment. *Seminars in Arthritis and Rheumatism.* 2013;43:178-86.

[115] J Pijpe, GW van Imhoff, FK Spijkervet, JL Roodenburg, GJ Wolbink, K Mansour, et al. Rituximab treatment in patients with primary Sjögren's syndrome: An open-label phase II study. *Arthritis & Rheumatism.* 2005;52: 2740-50.

[116] F Carubbi, P Cipriani, A Marrelli, P Benedetto, P Ruscitti, O Berardicurti, et al. Efficacy and safety of rituximab treatment in early primary Sjögren's syndrome: a prospective, multi-center, follow-up study. *Arthritis Research & Therapy.* 2013;15(5):R172.

[117] TR Reksten, MV Jonsson, EA Szyszko, JG Brun, R Jonsson, KA Brokstad. Cytokine and autoantibody profiling related to histopathological features in primary Sjögren's syndrome. *Rheumatology* (Oxford). 2009;48:1102 - 6.

[118] KB Norheim, E Harboe, LG Gøransson, R Omdal. Interleukin-1 inhibition and fatigue in primary Sjögren's syndrome--a double blind, randomised clinical trial. *PLoS One*. 2012;7(1):e30123.

[119] U Båve, G Nordmark, T Lövgren, J Rönnelid, S Cajander, ML Eloranta, et al. Activation of the type I interferon system in primary Sjögren's syndrome: a possible etiopathogenic mechanism. *Arthritis and Rheumatism* 2005;52(4):1185-95.

[120] N Roescher, PP Tak, GG Illei. Cytokines in Sjogren's syndrome: potential therapeutic targets. *Annals of the Rheumatic Diseases* 2010;69(6):945-8.

In: Sjögren's Syndrome
Editor: Eduardo M. Hernandez
ISBN: 978-1-63117-859-7


*Chapter III*

# Sjögren's Syndrome Symptoms and Diagnosis

***Antonio Bascones-Martínez[1,*], Elena Ruiz-Capillas, D.D.S.[2], Cristina Bascones-Ilundain, D.D.S., Ph.D.[3] and Virginia Garcia Garcia, D.D.S., Ph.D.[4]***

[1]Professor and Chairman of Oral Medicine and Periodontology. Faculty of Dentistry, Complutense University of Madrid, Madrid, Spain
[2]Expert in Periodontology. Faculty of Dentistry, Complutense University of Madrid, Madrid, Spain
[3]Associate Professor, Faculty of Dentistry, Complutense University of Madrid, Madrid, Spain
[4]Master in Periodontolgy, Faculty of Dentistry, Complutense University of Madrid, Madrid, Spain

## Abstract

Sjögren's syndrome (SS) is a multi-system exocrinopathy. Its etiology remains unknown and it has an autoimmune pathogenesis. Although SS has been reported in young children and men, it is more frequent in middle-aged women, with a sex ratio of 9:1. SS may occur

* Correspondence: antbasco@odon.ucm.es (*A. Bascones-Martínez).

alone, defined as primary SS, or in association with another autoimmune disease, defined as secondary SS. SS has a wide variety of glandular and extra-glandular manifestations affecting almost every organ. Despite its apparently inoffensive initial manifestations, SS can become a disabling and potentially life-threatening disease. Glandular manifestations vary according to the gland in question. The best predictor for SS is dry mouth (xerostomia), the most common SS symptom, followed by dry eyes. The low salivary flow increases susceptibility to bacterial and fungal diseases and often results in oral candidiasis. Dry eye (keratoconjunctivitissicca) is the most common ocular symptom. The main systemic manifestations are fatigue, dry airways, dry skin, dry vagina, dyspepsia, peripheral neuropathies, and autoimmune thyroiditis. Lymphoma, mostly of mucosa-associated lymphoid tissue type, is a characteristic but unusual feature that appears in approximately 5% of SS patients. The multiple manifestations of the syndrome and its insidious onset hamper its diagnosis. Besides the above symptoms, some objective signs are measured to make the definitive diagnosis of SS, using: ocular tests, notably Schirmer's I test and/or the Rose Bengal score; labial salivary gland biopsy, for assessing focal sialadenitis; scintigraphy, sialography, or unstimulated salivary flow, for evaluation of salivary gland involvement; and tests to detect the presence of Ro/SSA and/or La/SSB autoantibodies in serum.

# Introduction

Sjögren's syndrome (SS) is a multi-system exocrinopathy of unknown etiology with an autoimmune pathogenesis. The syndrome is frequently described as a disease of middle-aged women (40-50 years old) [1, 2], with a sex ratio of 9:1, similar to that of systemic lupus erythematosus (SLE) [3, 4] although it has also been reported in young children [5-7] and men [8, 9]. SS is the second most common autoimmune rheumatic disease, with an estimated prevalence ranging from 0.1 to 4.8% [10].

Sjögren's syndrome may occur alone, defined as primary Sjögren's syndrome (pSS), or in association with another defined autoimmune disease, such as rheumatoid arthritis (RA), systemic lupus erythematosus (SLE), or scleroderma, observed in half of SS cases and defined as secondary SS [11].

The salivary and lacrimal glands are the principal targets of a supposedly T and B cell-mediated chronic inflammation that destroys the glandular parenchyma. Exocrine glands in the vagina, skin, pancreas, and respiratory and gastrointestinal systems can also be affected, and extra-glandular processes in SS can involve the joints, liver, kidneys, and central nervous system (CNS).

The cardinal manifestation of SS is dryness leading to dry eyes (keratoconjunctivitissicca) and mouth (xerostomia), but it also presents a wide variety of systemic manifestations. Although the initial symptoms of SS may seem innocuous, SS can progress to a disabling and potentially life-threatening malignancy.

As described by Hatron [12], there are two forms of the disease:

- An "epithelial" form, limited to dryness symptoms. It is often associated with arthralgia, myalgia, and fatigue.
- An "extra-epithelial" form, with recurrent parotid inflammation and more systemic manifestations. It is characterized by the presence of hypergammaglobulinemia and cryoglobulinemia and a higher frequency of anti-SSA and SSB antibodies with lower complement levels. It carries a higher risk of lymphoma and other severe complications.

The multiple manifestations of the syndrome and its insidious onset complicate the diagnosis. Thus, SS patients commonly remain undiagnosed (in more than a half of the cases) or are diagnosed years after the onset of symptoms. An early and accurate diagnosis of the disease is essential to prevent many of its associated complications or ensure their timely treatment, including serious systemic complications such as malignant lymphoma and interstitial lung disease. The correct diagnosis of SS depends on recognizing its clinical manifestations, ruling out alternatives in the differential diagnosis, and distinguishing between primary and secondary SS.

## Oral Symptoms

Xerostomia, the symptom of dry mouth, is commonly related to a low salivary rate (hyposalivation), mainly when the unstimulated salivary flow falls below 50% of normal values. However, xerostomia in SS patients has been more associated with changes in the quality of salivary mucins rather than in the quantity of salivary flow [13]. These patients are also susceptible to alterations in soft and hard tissues [14].

In the early stages of SS, salivary flow can still be relatively normal but there can be a loss of salivary function. The mouth may appear moist, because the inflammation has not yet destroyed the salivary glands to a significant degree; however, as the disease progresses, the usual pooling of saliva in the floor of the mouth disappears, and lines of contact can be observed between frothy saliva and oral soft tissue. In advanced disease, the oral mucosa appears dry, pale, and glazed and tends to form fine mucosal wrinkles, and the lips are cracked and atrophic; the surface of the tongue typically becomes red and lobulated, with partial or complete depapillation.

Saliva plays an essential role in oral microbiota because it contains defensins, proteases, histatins, and lysozyme among others. Several studies have demonstrated modifications in the oral microbial composition of individuals with hyposalivation [15, 16]. Although the total salivary bacterial count was found to be similar between SS patients and controls [17], a high bacterial count of species such as *Lactobacillus acidophilus*, *Streptococcus mutans* [18] and *Candida albicans* was reported. Hence, the plaque had a more cariogenic and acidophilic profile in the patients than in the controls, elevating the risk of caries. The increased susceptibility of SS patients to bacterial and fungal diseases has been attributed to the absence of the buffer effect of saliva [19]. These features correlate with a higher incidence of infectious diseases such as caries and candidiasis [14].

A low salivary flow is associated with increased plaque accumulation and reduced sugar clearance, which together lead to increased levels of carious lesions at sites favoring the retention of dental plaque (e.g., next to dental fillings or along the gingival margin of root surfaces) as well as at other sites (e.g., lingual, incisal, and cuspal tooth surfaces) [14].

The elevated *Candida albicans* count of SS patients means that oral candidiasis develops in 30-70% of them, despite good oral hygiene. They are also at higher risk of developing fungal lesions at the corners of the mouth (angular cheilitis). Xerostomia is not usually associated with pain; therefore, examinations for signs of angular cheilitis or oral candidiasis should be conducted in cases of sudden pain onset [20].

Patients with SS have also been reported to have an increased risk of periodontal disease, but this association is less firmly established than that with dental caries. The available evidence suggests that the periodontal status of SS patients is similar to that of controls and there is no need for special periodontal care [21, 22].

Although the presenting symptoms of SS are frequently those of xerostomia, the patient may complain of dysphagia [23], increased water intake, soreness, nocturnal discomfort, difficulties in denture control [24], adherence of food to buccal surfaces or fissuring of the tongue, rather than of oral dryness. The taste buds may be abnormal and their number decreased, resembling those of patients with idiopathic hypogeusia, and SS patients may note an unpleasant taste. Hypersensitivity of the oral mucosa and burning sensations are also frequent. Some patients may have difficulties with speech, making a "clicking" sound because of the tongue sticking to the palate in the absence of moisture [25].

Enlargement of salivary glands, frequently of the parotid gland, is observed in up to 50% of SS patients and is one of the early manifestations of juvenile disease. The swelling is painless and can be chronic or episodic and unilateral or bilateral. Among out-patients, SS is the most frequent underlying cause of acute bacterial sialadenitis, usually staphylococcal or pneumococcal. Affected patients typically report acute pain, trismus, and a tender swelling of the salivary gland. Regional lymph nodes may be enlarged and tender, and there may be fever and malaise in severe cases [25]. A lymphoma should be ruled out if there is a sudden increase in size with pain and a hard consistency.

## Ocular Manifestations

The characteristic ophthalmologic finding in Sjögren syndrome is dry eye: keratoconjunctivitissicca (KCS) from decreased lacrimal secretion, due to destruction of the lacrimal glands [26]. In severe cases, patients may have strings of mucous filaments attached to the cornea. Ocular complications can also include corneal ulceration or perforation.

Eye dryness isparticularly marked in the morning, because there is no tear restoration during sleep time. Although the eyes generally have a normal appearance, manifestations of dry eye include sensations of itching, grittiness (a 'sandy' feeling), or soreness [27]. Intolerance to contact lenses may be an initial symptom, probably due to corneal edema. This syndrome also increases photosensitivity and may oblige some patients to wear sunglasses permanently. Other signs and symptoms may include blurred vision (improves after blinking), erythema, eye fatigue (frequently at the end of the day), eye discharges, and the sensation of a film across the visual field [28]. These symptoms may be exacerbated by environmental dryness generated in some climates or by excessive air-conditioning use, smoke, anxiety, depression, or anticholinergic drugs [25].

In severe cases, ocular complications can include corneal erosions that sometimes lead to corneal ulceration or, more rarely, to perforation, filamentary keratitis, marked by mucus filaments that adhere to damaged areas of the corneal surface; conjunctivitis due to *Staphylococcus aureus* infection, vascularization, opacification, eyelid infections, dilation of the bulbar conjunctival vessels and, rarely, perforation [25]. Lacrimal gland swelling is infrequent and a mucosa-associated lymphoid tissue (MALT) lymphoma should be ruled out in such cases [29].

## Gynecological Features

In female patients with SS, desiccation of the vagina and vulva may result in dyspareunia, pruritus and increased frequency of vaginal candidiasis [30], as well as polyuria, nocturia, and urge incontinence due to irritable bladder. A study of 169 female SS patients reported vaginal symptoms in 26% [29], while Marchesoni et al. [31] observed dyspareunia in 61% of SS patients *versus*39% of women in the control group and vaginal dryness in 52% of patients *versus* 33% of controls. However, Skoupoli et al. [32] found no difference in fertility, parity, or reproductive success between 51 women with pSS and 57 healthy controls; vaginal atrophy and reduced cervical mucus production were correlated with age and menopause but not with any clinical or serologic manifestation of the syndrome.

Dyspareunia was observed in 40% of the pre-menopausal patients in comparison to 3% of controls, although the etiology of the dyspareunia was evident in half of the patents (trauma or inflammation) and unrelated to the pSS. It has been suggested that these findings may be related not only to an underlying autoimmune effect of SS but also to the stress of suffering from a chronic illness, which tends to reduce vaginal moisture [31].

## Respiratory Involvement

The impairment and destruction of exocrine glands in SS may involve the respiratory tract. The lesions can be related either to sicca symptoms (glandular involvement) or to cell infiltrate (extraglandular involvement). The reported frequency of respiratory symptoms in SS patients ranges widely from 9 to 75%; although a narrower range of 9-12% was found when only clinically significant manifestations were considered [33, 34]. SS may be misdiagnosed as late-onset asthma, because the syndrome sometimes mimics non-allergic asthma in its early stage [12].

The respiratory tract is a frequent localization of these lesions. The reduction or disappearance of glandular secretions in the airway can lead to xerotrachea, producing a decrease in mucociliary clearance, which may hamper expectoration and thereby favor infections. This symptom also causes dryness of the nose, throat, and trachea, resulting in persistent hoarseness and a chronic nonproductive cough. Around half of patients with SS report a dry cough during the day and night that impairs their quality of life [35]. Recurrent respiratory infections (bronchitis, pneumonia) are associated with airway dysfunction in 20% of SS patients. The predilection of SS for the bronchial tree is confirmed by the high frequency of radiological patterns related to airway disease [12].

Interstitial lung disease affects 8-38% of SSpatients, with a wide variety of manifestations ranging from an absence of symptoms to dyspnea, cough and crackles [11]. Severe interstitial disease in SS is rare [35]. Interstitial lung disease or pleural involvement are seldom the earliest manifestation of the disease [36].

## Cutaneous Manifestations

Cutaneous manifestations of SS include dry skin, immunologic inflammatory conditions, e.g., vasculitis, and other associated skin conditions. Dry skin is observed in around 50% of SS patients, although it is unclear whether it is attributable to infiltrations of the eccrine or sebaceous glands or to dysfunctional sweating [26].

Vascular findings in SS include purpura, leukocytoclastic vasculitis, and urticarial vasculitis, frequently on the legs. A recent study found vasculitis in 10% of SS patients [37], while a study by Kyle et al. [38] of a large cohort of patients with hyperglobulinemic purpura reported that around half of them had SS. Purpura has also been associated with CNS [39] or pulmonary involvement [40]. Other authors have demonstrated that cutaneous purpura is associated with lymphoma development and mortality in SS patients [32, 41]. Raynaud's phenomenon is another common sign of SS, with a prevalence of around 30%, and it can appear many years before diagnosis of the disease [37, 42, 43].

Patients with pSS may also present with a wide range of non-vasculitic lesions, including eyelid dermatitis, pruritus, erythema annulare, vitiligo, subcutaneous amyloidanetoderma, alopecia, and cutaneous lymphomas, while the presence of anetoderma has been associated with B-cell lymphomas [44].

One of the most characteristic findings is annular erythema, which is clinically identical to that observed in patients with subacute cutaneous lupus erythematosus (SCLE), suggesting that the latter group and pSS patients share a common origin [11].

## Gastrointestinal Manifestations

Gastrointestinal manifestations include dysphagia, which is partly due to xerostomia but may also be causedby motility abnormalities, lower pressure of the esophageal sphincter and/or reduced contractility [28]. Patients also complain of dyspepsia, nausea, and epigastric pain, which can be associated with gastritis, reduced acid production, and antiparietal cell antibodies, also known as autoimmune gastritis [29].

Hyposalivation contributes to gastrointestinal involvement because gastric acid reflux is neutralized by saliva, which has an alkaline pH; hence, SS patients may be predisposed to gastroesophageal reflux, while reflux into the trachea can mimic upper respiratory tract infection in some cases [45].

Patients with gastritis should be examined for *Helicobacter pylori*, especially given its association with MALT lymphoma in SS patients [46]. Slight atrophic changes were found to be more frequent in SS patients than in controls, but severe mucosal atrophy was uncommon [47].

Volter et al. [48] evaluated esophageal function and gastroesophageal reflux in 21 SS patients, 100% of whom evidenced xerostomia, 33% dysphagia, and 62% heartburn, with no differences between those with primary and secondary SS. They concluded that the early and accurate diagnosis of gastroesophageal reflux is essential to identify SS patients at risk of acidic reflux, especially given the lower acid-clearance capacity of the esophagus due to hyposalivation.

## Fatigue

Fatigue is one of the most frequent symptoms in pSS patients, appearing in around 70% of cases [49], and it can sometimes be the most disabling manifestation [50]. Although instruments for fatigue assessment are inadequate and there has been little research, it appears that physical and somatic rather than mental aspects of fatigue are more severely and frequently involved in pSS [51].

The pathogenesis of fatigue is poorly understood, and multiple factors have been implicated. Barendregt et al. [50] compared fatigue in relation to depression, blood pressure, and plasma catecholamines among 49 pSS patients, 32 healthy controls, and 44 RA patients. Fatigue was greater in SS patients than in controls for all studied dimensions and the difference remained significant for physical fatigue, general fatigue, and reduced activity after controlling for depression. A negative correlation was found between noradrenaline levels and general fatigue in the SS patients.

Another study [52] investigated the association between fatigue severity and other clinical features in 94 pSS subjects with the aim of identifying contributing factors. Abnormal fatigue was present in 67% of the patients and was most strongly associated with pain, helplessness, and depression. They found that psychosocial factors only partially explained the fatigue, concluding that fatigue is related to depression but that depression is not the primary cause of fatigue in pSS.

## Renal Involvement

Renal disease has been reported in 4.2% of pSS patients in one study [53] and 67% in another [54]. The wide discrepancy in prevalence data has been attributed to differences in diagnostic criteria and study design [55]. Tubulointerstitial nephritis is the most frequent kidney manifestation. The tubular damage may result in distal renal tubular acidosis, which sometimes lead to compromised renal function, proteinuria, kidney stones, hypokalemia, hypophosphatemia, polyuria, and/ornephrogenic diabetes insipidus [11]. Glomerulonephritis is less frequent, being a late sign, but may produce hypertension or proteinuria and is related to higher morbidity and mortality rates. The difference between tubular *versus* glomerular renal disease has major prognostic implications for SS patients [25, 55, 56].

## Muscular Involvement

Muscular manifestations and symptoms of weakness are also frequent [26]. Lindvall et al. [57] described myalgia in around 30% of patients with pSS, finding that 27% of the patients fulfilled diagnostic criteria for fibromyalgia, similar to the report by Ostuni et al. [58] of fibromyalgia in 22% of pSS patients. About 4% of the patients are found to have polymyositis [29].

## Neurological Manifestations

Neurological complications are observed in around 20% of pSS patients and can be inaugural; they include peripheral and central nervous system manifestations, which may both be related to a vasculitic process [26, 59].

The prevalence of peripheral neuropathy in SS patients varies from 20 to 60% and can precede diagnosis of the syndrome (29, 60). Pure sensory neuropathy (PSN) is the most common type and is considered a characteristic neurological feature of SS [11, 26]; patients with this neuropathyhave symmetrical and distal paresthesias, neuropathic pain, and burning foot sensations, while clinical examination shows reduced or absent deep tendon reflexes [59].

Cranial nerves may also be impaired. The cochlear nerve is frequently involved, resulting in hearing loss and vestibular symptoms. Sensory trigeminal and facial nerve disorders are also commonly reported [60]. Other possible neurological manifestations in SS include painful sensory neuropathy, multiple mononeuropathy, polyradiculopathy, and autonomic neuropathy [29].

Although CNS involvement was considered a frequent extraglandular manifestation of SS in earlier studies, more recent studies of large series have revealed that symptomatic CNS involvement is not so common [11]. CNS manifestations include diffuse brain lesions, spinal cord involvement, subacute aseptic meningitis, chorea, and optic neuritis, among others. Estimates of the prevalence of these manifestations range widely from 8% to 40% [29].

Primary SS patients frequently evidence cognitive changes with poor concentration and memory [29, 59], including executive dysfunction, visuospatial disorders and long- or short-term memory deficits, irrespective of the presence of depressive disorders [59]. Although these symptoms are often not reported by patients, they can be detected by formal cognitive testing [26].

# Psychiatric Manifestations

Psychiatric disorders, including depression and anxiety, have been frequently reported in SS patients. The increased frequency indicates that they might be attributable to the underlying process instead of being a response to the stress of having an autoimmune disorder. These manifestations often appear before the syndrome has been diagnosed [26].

# Endocrine Involvement

Around 20-45% [25, 49] of patients with pSS develop autoimmune thyroiditis, and more than 50% have subclinical hypothyroidism. Some studies have reported that autoimmune thyroiditis is nine-fold more prevalent in SS patients.

Conversely, SS is 10-fold more prevalent among patients with than without autoimmune thyroid disease [1]. Hashimoto's thyroiditis is the most frequent manifestation, followed by Graves' disease [49]. Autoantibodies against thyroid peroxidase (anti-TPO) and thyroglobulin (anti-TG) may indicate a propensity to develop thyroid disease [61].

# Articular Manifestations

Articular involvement is reported in 45-55% of patients with SS [29, 62], although it appears to be less frequent in elderly patients. Arthropathy sometimes appears before SS. Articular pain (arthralgia) and polyarthropathy are the most common symptoms [25, 29] and largely involve peripheral joints.

Arthralgias have been described in 53% of SS patients, with a similar symmetric distribution and appearance to those in RA or SLE [26]. Polyarthropathy in SS can be symmetrical or asymmetrical, with an intermittentnon-erosive pattern that affects both small and large joints. Joint deformity synovitis and mild erosions are infrequent, while a transient non-erosive arthritis similar to that in SLE can be observed [25, 29]. The presence of an asymmetric swollen joint may indicate an additional disease, such as crystalline or infectious arthropathy [26].

Fauchais et al. [62] found articular involvement in 188 out of 419 (45%) patients with pSS, of whom 17% presented with these manifestations before the SS diagnosis. The authors concluded that articular manifestations are frequent in pSS patients and are associated with a plurisystemic involvement of the syndrome, although they are usually mild.

## Lymphoma

Lymphomas are a characteristic but unusual feature of SS, observed in around 5% of patients [27, 63]. Conversely, patients with SS have a20- to 40-fold higher risk of lymphoma than those without, a much greater risk than reported for patients with other autoimmune diseases [26, 64], while malignant non-Hodgkin's lymphoma is considered to be the most severe SS complication [63]. Ioannidis et al. [41] found that 20% of the mortality in patients with pSS was attributable to lymphoma. There have also been reports of the association of lymphoma in SS patients with various infectious agents, including helicobacter pylori, human herpes virus, and Epstein-Barr virus [26].

In 1999, Voulgarelis et al. [63] published a multicenter study designed by the European Concerted Action on SS that included 33 patients with pSS who developed malignant non-Hodgkin lymphoma. Lymphoproliferative neoplasms in these patients were almost exclusively of B cell lineage and were mostly MALT lymphomas, localized in the marginal zone and affecting the salivary glands; they also showed extranodal involvement. Lymphadenopathy, vasculitis, peripheral nerve involvement, fever, anemia, and lymphopenia were also significantly more frequent than in the general population of SS patients. The patients with lymphoma had a significantly worse survival rate.

Although the manifestations are non-specific, the development of a lymphoma may be indicated by the presence of persistently enlarged parotid or regional or generalized lymphadenopathy, hepatosplenomegaly, pulmonary infiltrates, and/or vasculitis [26, 64], especially when accompanied by falling hematocrit values, a high sedimentation rate, monoclonal cryoglobulinemia [26] or low complement levels of C4 and C3 [64]. Low C4 and C3 levels were found to be the only independent risk factor, and hypocomplementemia was related to a decreased survival in these patients [65].

## Secondary SS

This term is used to described patients suffering from another autoimmune disease concomitant with Sjögren's syndrome. RA is the most common disease in secondary SS. A persistent synovitis on metacarpophalangeal joints in pSS should suggest RA. Usually, but not always, SS appears some years later than the RA diagnosis [11]. These patients generally develop amore severe disease with increased extra-articular manifestations, including vasculitis. In SLE, however, patients with SS have a lower frequency of glomerulonephritis and a relatively good prognosis. Primary biliary cirrhosis and scleroderma, although rare, are frequently complicated by SS. Polymyositis, chronic active hepatitis, mixed connective tissue disease, and Hashimoto's thyroiditis have also been described in association with Sjögren's syndrome [64].

# Diagnosis

## Salivary Tests

Xerostomia is one of the cardinal manifestations of SS, and the accessibility of saliva supports the use of sialometry and sialochemistry in the diagnosis of the disease [66]. The objective demonstration of this xerostomia by measuring salivary flow (sialometry) should be the first step in the examination of patients suspected of SS. The collection and analysis of whole saliva is the most used technique for sialometry, despite its inaccurate and impure nature. The unstimulated whole saliva is collected during 15 min, and the measurement is considered positive when <1.5 ml is cumulated. This test has a sensitivity of 56.1% and an 80.7% of specificity for SS diagnosis [11, 64].

Sialochemical analysis allows the evaluation of a wide spectrum of salivary components, including calcium, sodium, chloride, urea, phosphate, amylase, lactoferrin, mucin and total protein. Kalk et al. [66] found significant differences in flow rates and salivary composition between healthy controls and SS patients, with the latter having lower sublingual/submandibular flow rates and an altered salivary composition. They concluded that the most accurate diagnostic test for SS is a combination of the stimulated sublingual/submandibular flow rate with parotid sodium and chloride concentrations.

Scintigraphy with 99m Tc-pertechnate is a key examination in the study of salivary glands function, intravenously administering 10 millicuries of the ion. The typical finding in SS patients is a decreased uptake in response to stimulation of the parotid and submandibular salivary glands. The results is based on the stages described by Schall et al. [67]: grade I = normal function, grade II = mild damage, grade III = moderate involvement, and grade IV =

severe functional defect. This test offers high sensitivity in the hands of skilled personnel but has a weak specificity.

Parotid sialography is a radiologic technique that uses contrast to visualize the salivary ducts, but it has little utility in SS diagnosis. The test typically shows sialectasias in patients with xerostomy in contrast to the fine arborization seen in healthy subjects.

## Ocular Test

Rose Bengal is a dye with affinity for devitalized/dead cells and mucin, revealing injured areas and mucus particles. Its elevated affinity means that the dye remains in the eye for a long time, and an anesthetic solution should be applied during its utilization to avoid irritation. The patient is asked to blink after receiving the dye, and the number of colored points is then counted in three regions of the ocular surface, which are scored on a scale of 0 – 3: 0= no points, 1= few separated points, 2= numerous separated points, and 3= confluent points. The test is considered positive if the sum of the score for the three regions is >4.

Another essential ocular test is the Schirmer test I, in which What man no. 41filter paper is anchored to the outer third of the lower eyelid. Patients then close their eyes and maintain the paper in this position for five minutes. The amount of paper moistened is measured in millimeters, with values below 10 mm indicating a deficiency in tear production. This test has a high specificity [68]. Lissamine green has the same features as Rose Bengaldye but is much less irritating. A score between 0-3 is given according to the staining of the nasal and temporal bulbar conjunctivae. Sodium fluorescein stains areas with loss of epithelial cells. The patient blinks after application of the dye and the eye is observed under cobalt blue filter. Superficial lesions fluoresce in a pale yellow color, while deeper lesions appear bright green. The fluorescent cornea is scored on a scale from 0 to 6. The ocular staining score (OSS) is the sum of the scores for fluorescein staining and for lissamine green, yielding a total score ranging from 0–12 [69].

## Serologic Tests

One of the main features of autoimmunity is the presence of autoantibodies. Anti-Ro antibodies bind to two related proteins attached to the RNA in the cytoplasm human. The pathogenetic role of anti-Ro is not known.

Anti-Roprevalence varies between 40-80% in pSS, and antibodies are also observed in secondary SS. Anti-La antibodies recognize a nuclear phosphoprotein that functions as an auxiliary factor in the terminal phase of transcription by inducing conformational changes in the RNA polymerase III [11]. The presence of anti-La antibodies varies between 30 and 60%. The utilization of distinct detection methods accounts for this wide range in estimated prevalence, which is improved by the application of immunoenzymatic methods (ELISA) [64]. The antibody levels do not significantly change over the course of the disease [11].

Anti-Ro antibodies are commonly present in the absence of anti-La reactivity. In contrast, Anti-La is always accompanied by anti-Ro, reflecting the physical association of these molecules in Ro/La ribonucleoprotein particles [64]. Positive serology is associated with a high frequency of palpablepurpura, leukopenia, lymphopenia, and hypergammaglobulinemia, and with more severe glandular disease.

## Labial Salivary Gland Biopsy

At present, biopsy of the major salivary glands is not considered for the study of patients with xerostomia, only being indicated in the presence of a mass or suspected tumor. Labial salivary gland biopsy plays an important role in establishing the diagnosis of SS. It allows differentiation between glandular involution caused by aging and the infiltration of salivary glands by SS, sarcoidosis, or even lymphoma. It is performed on an outpatient basis in clinically intact mucosa with infiltrating anesthesia between the labial commissure and middle of the lower lip. A horizontal incision of 1.5-2 cm is made parallel to the vermilion border in the middle of the lower lip, penetrating the epithelium, followed by the blunt dissection of at least five lobes. In the biopsy evaluation, an inflammatory focus is defined as an accumulation of $\geq$ 50 mononuclear leukocytes per4 $mm^2$ [70]. According to the AECG criteria [71], a biopsy is positive with a focus score >1 per 4 $mm^2$. The specificity of a positive labial salivary gland biopsy for pSSis86.2% and the sensitivity is 82.4%.

## Diagnostic Criteria

Since 1965, 12 different criteria for the diagnosis and classification of Sjögren's syndrome have published. In 1993, preliminary European criteria

[72], consisting of both objective and subjective criteria, were proposed and widely accepted. They were revised in 2002 by the American-European Consensus Group (AECG) [71], which proposed another classification with stricter and more precise requirements (Table 1). The AECG criteria have been found to offer improved specificity and have been considered the gold standard for over a decade. They have been the basis for the development of disease activity and disease damage scores and used in more than 1300 papers. However, they have been criticized for including subjective elements and the possibility of alternate diagnostic tests that are not fully equivalent.

**Table 1. Classification criteria for Sjögren's syndrome proposed by the AECG [71]**

| |
|---|
| *I. Ocular symptoms* (positive response to at least one of the following questions)<br>- Have you had daily, persistent, troublesome dry eyes for more than 3 months?<br>- Do you have a recurrent sensation of sand or gravel in the eyes?<br>- Do you use tear substitutes more than 3 times a day? |
| *II. Oral symptoms* (positive response to at least one of the following questions)<br>- Have you had a daily feeling of dry mouth for more than 3 months?<br>- Have you had recurrently or persistently swollen salivary glands as an adult?<br>- Do you frequently drink liquids to aid in swallowing dry food? |
| *III. Ocular objective signs* (positive result for at least one of the following tests)<br>- Schirmer's I test, performed without anesthesia (<5 mm in 5 minutes)<br>- Rose Bengal score or other ocular dye score (>4 according to van Bijsterveld's scoring system) |
| *IV. Histopathology*<br>Focal lymphocytic sialoadenitis in minor salivary glands, evaluated by an expert histopathologist, with a focus score >1 |
| *V. Salivary gland objective involvement* (positive result for at least one of the following tests)<br>- Unstimulated whole salivary flow (<1.5 ml in 15 minutes)<br>- Parotid sialography showing the presence of diffuse sialectasias, without evidence of obstruction in the major ducts<br>- Salivary scintigraphy showing delayed uptake, reduced concentration and/or delayed excretion of tracer |
| *VI. Autoantibodies* (presence in the serum of the following autoantibodies)<br>Antibodies to Ro(SSA) or La(SSB) antigens, or both |
| *Rules for classification*<br>For primary SS: patients without any potentially associated disease<br>- The presence of any 4 of the 6 items, as long as either histopathology or serology is positive<br>- The presence of any 3 of the 4 objective criteria items (items III to VI)<br>- The classification tree procedure represents a valid alternative classification method, although it should be more properly used in clinical-epidemiological survey<br>For s**econdary SS:** patients with a potentially associated disease<br>- The presence of item I or II plus any 2 from among items III, IV, and V<br>*Exclusion criteria:* past head and neck radiation treatment, hepatitis C infection, AIDS, pre-existing lymphoma, sarcoidosis, graft versus host disease, use of anticholinergic drugs (for a shorter time than 4-fold the half-life of the drug). |

**Table 2. ACR Classification Criteria for Sjögren's Syndrome [69]**

| |
|---|
| *Classification rules:* patients must meet at least 2 of the following 3 objective features:<br>1. Positive serum anti-SSA/Ro and/or anti-SSB/La or (positive rheumatoid factor and ANA titer ≥1:320)<br>2. Labial salivary gland biopsy exhibiting focal lymphocytic sialadenitis with a focus score ≥1 focus/4 $mm^2$<br>3. Keratoconjunctivitissicca with ocular staining score ≥3 (assuming that individual is not currently using daily eye drops for glaucoma and has not had corneal surgery or cosmetic eyelid surgery in the last 5 years)<br><br>Patients with rheumatoid arthritis, systemic lupus erythematosus, scleroderma, or other connective tissue disease were excluded. |
| *Exclusion criteria*<br>History of head and neck radiation treatment<br>Hepatitis C infection<br>Acquired immunodeficiency syndrome<br>Sarcoidosis<br>Amyloidosis<br>Graft versus host disease<br>IgG4-related disease |

In 2012, in an attempt to overcome these shortcomings, the Sjögren's International Collaborative Clinical Alliance (SICCA-ACR) [69] published another diagnostic system based solely on objective criteria that did not require the presence of dry eyes or mouth for the diagnosis (Table 2). This new system was provisionally adopted by the American College of Rheumatology (ACR). Rasmussen et al. [73] conducted a study in a well-characterized sicca cohort comparing the AECG and the SICCA-ACR classification criteria for SS and concluded that the two sets yielded concordant results in the majority of cases. Neither classification is perfect, but they may offer the opportunity for developing a more robust classification for future use [74].

# Conclusion

Sjögren's syndrome is a common autoimmune disease that compromises the health of patients at almost every level (Table 3). The multiple manifestations of SS and its insidious onset complicate the diagnosis.

**Table 3. Manifestations of Sjögren syndrome**

| | |
|---|---|
| **Oral** | |
| • xerostomia<br>• caries<br>• candidiasis<br>• dysphagia<br>• increased water intake<br>• soreness<br>• enlarged glands | • difficulties in controlling dentures<br>• adherence of food to buccal surfaces<br>• fissured tongue.<br>• abnormal taste<br>• burning sensations of the oral mucosa<br>• difficulties with speech |
| Ocular | |
| • keratoconjunctivitissicca<br>• itching, grittiness, soreness<br>• intolerance to contact lenses<br>• photosensitivity<br>• sensation of a film across the visual field | • blurred vision<br>• erythema<br>• eye fatigue<br>• discharge<br>• erosions, ulcerations, perforations |
| Gynecological | |
| • vaginal dryness<br>• dyspareunia<br>• pruritus<br>• candidiasis | • polyuria<br>• nocturia<br>• incontinence |
| Respiratory | |
| • xerotrachea<br>• dry nose and throat<br>• infections (bronchitis, pneumonia) | • hoarseness<br>• chronic, nonproductive cough<br>• interstitial lung disease |
| Cutaneous | |
| • dry skin<br>• vasculitis<br>• purpura<br>• Raynaud's phenomenon<br>• eyelid dermatitis<br>• pruritus | • vitíligo<br>• subcutaneous amyloidanetoderma<br>• alopecia<br>• cutaneous lymphomas<br>• anetoderma<br>• erythema annulare |
| Gastrointestinal | |
| • dysphagia<br>• dyspepsia, nausea and epigastric pain | • gastroesophageal reflux<br>• autoimmune gastritis |
| Fatigue | |
| Renal | |
| • Tubulointerstitial nephritis<br>• distal renal tubular acidosis<br>• proteinuria<br>• kidney stones | • hypokalemia<br>• hypophosphatemia<br>• polyuria<br>• diabetes insipidus |
| Muscular | |
| • myalgias<br>• fybromyalgias | • polymyositis |
| Neurological | |

| Oral | |
|---|---|
| • pure sensory neuropathy<br>• painful sensory neuropathy<br>• multiple mononeuropathy<br>• polyradiculopathy<br>• autonomic neuropathy<br>• paresthesias<br>• neuropathic pain | • burning feet sensations<br>• diffuse brain lesions,<br>• spinal cord involvement<br>• subacute aseptic meningitis,<br>• chorea<br>• optic neuritis<br>• cognitive disorders |
| Psychiatric | |
| • depression | • anxiety |
| Endocrinal | |
| • autoimmune thyroiditis | |
| Articular | |
| • arthralgia | • polyarthropathy |
| Lymphoma | |
| • MALT | |

Al-Hashimi et al. [1] investigated the predictive value of numerous different manifestations by comparing the clinical profiles of 169 SS patients with those of 44 healthy controls. They found that the combined presence of dry mouth, sore mouth, and dry eyes correctly classified almost all individuals. Their results suggest that the diagnosis of SS may be improved by using a questionnaire to gather different symptoms. Numerous authors have proposed sets of SS criteria in attempts to resolve the difficulties in diagnosing SS. Two scientifically validated criteria are currently available: American-European Consensus Group criteria, used for more than a decade; and the recently proposed and validated American College of Rheumatology criteria. These are not without limitations but may provide the basis for an update and improvement of diagnostic criteria for this syndrome.

## References

[1] Al-Hashimi I, Khuder S, Haghighat N, Zipp M. Frequency and predictive value of the clinical manifestations in Sjögren's syndrome. *Journal Of Oral Pathology & Medicine: Official Publication Of The International Association Of Oral Pathologists And The American Academy Of Oral Pathology*. 2001; 30(1):1-6.

[2] Scully C. Sjögren's syndrome: clinical and laboratory features, immunopathogenesis, and management. *Oral surgery, oral medicine, and oral pathology*. 1986; 62(5):510-23.

[3] Bowman SJ, Ibrahim GH, Holmes G, Hamburger J, Ainsworth JR. Estimating the prevalence among Caucasian women of primary Sjögren's syndrome in two general practices in Birmingham, UK. *Scandinavian journal of rheumatology*. 2004; 33(1):39-43.

[4] Fox RI, Tornwall J, Michelson P. Current issues in the diagnosis and treatment of Sjögren's syndrome. *Current opinion in rheumatology*. 1999; 11(5):364-71.

[5] Anaya JM, Ogawa N, Talal N. Sjögren's syndrome in childhood. *The Journal of rheumatology*. 1995; 22(6):1152-8.

[6] Flaitz CM. Parotitis as the initial sign of juvenile Sjogren's syndrome. *Pediatric dentistry*. 2001; 23(2):140-2.

[7] Hearth-Holmes M, Baethge BA, Abreo F, Wolf RE. Autoimmune exocrinopathy presenting as recurrent parotitis of childhood. *Archives of Otolaryngology--Head & Neck Surgery*. 1993; 119(3):347-9.

[8] Anaya JM, Liu GT, D'Souza E, Ogawa N, Luan X, Talal N. Primary Sjögren's syndrome in men. *Annals of the Rheumatic Diseases*. 1995; 54(9):748-51.

[9] Horvath IF, Szodoray P, Zeher M. Primary Sjögren's syndrome in men: clinical and immunological characteristic based on a large cohort of Hungarian patients. *Clinical rheumatology*. 2008; 27(12):1479-83.

[10] Delaleu N, Jonsson R, Koller MM. Sjogren's syndrome. *European journal of oral sciences*. 2005; 113(2):101-13.

[11] Anaya JM, Casals MR, Carrasco MG. *Síndrome de Sjögren*. Medellín, Colombia: Corporación para Investigaciones Biológicas; 2001.

[12] Hatron P-Y, Tillie-Leblond I, Launay D, Hachulla E, Fauchais AL, Wallaert B. *Pulmonary manifestations of Sjögren's syndrome*. Presse Médicale (Paris, France: 1983). 2011; 40(1):e49-e64.

[13] Alliende C, Kwon YJ, Brito M, Molina C, Aguilera S, Perez P, et al. Reduced sulfation of muc5b is linked to xerostomia in patients with Sjogren syndrome. *Ann. Rheum. Dis.* 2008; 67(10):1480-7.

[14] Gonzalez S, Sung H, Sepulveda D, Gonzalez M, Molina C. Oral manifestations and their treatment in Sjogren's syndrome. *Oral diseases*. 2014; 20(2):153-61.

[15] van Houte J. Role of micro-organisms in caries etiology. *Journal of dental research*. 1994; 73(3):672-81.

[16] Marsh PD, Keevil CW, McDermid AS, Williamson MI, Ellwood DC. Inhibition by the antimicrobial agent chlorhexidine of acid production and sugar transport in oral streptococcal bacteria. *Archives of oral biology*. 1983; 28(3):233-40.

[17] Lundstrom IM, Lindstrom FD. Subjective and clinical oral symptoms in patients with primary Sjogren's syndrome. *Clinical and experimental rheumatology.* 1995; 13(6):725-31.

[18] Almståhl A, Wikström M, Kroneld U. Microflora in oral ecosystems in primary Sjögren's syndrome. *The Journal of rheumatology.* 2001; 28(5): 1007-13.

[19] van der Reijden WA, Vissink A, Veerman EC, Amerongen AV. Treatment of oral dryness related complaints (xerostomia) in Sjogren's syndrome. *Ann. Rheum. Dis.* 1999; 58(8):465-74.

[20] Daniels TE. Evaluation, differential diagnosis, and treatment of xerostomia. *The Journal of rheumatology Supplement.* 2000; 61:6-10.

[21] Kuru B, McCullough MJ, Yilmaz S, Porter SR. Clinical and microbiological studies of periodontal disease in Sjogren syndrome patients. *Journal of clinical periodontology.* 2002; 29(2):92-102.

[22] Schiodt M, Christensen LB, Petersen PE, Thorn JJ. Periodontal disease in primary Sjogren's syndrome. *Oral diseases.* 2001; 7(2):106-8.

[23] Rhodus NL, Colby S, Moller K, Bereuter J. Quantitative assessment of dysphagia in patients with primary and secondary Sjogren's syndrome. *Oral surgery, oral medicine, oral pathology, oral radiology, and endodontics.* 1995; 79(3):305-10.

[24] Binon PP, Fowler CN. Implant-supported fixed prosthesis treatment of a patient with Sjogren's syndrome: a *clinical report. The* International journal of oral & maxillofacial implants. 1993; 8(1):54-8.

[25] Kassan SS, Moutsopoulos HM. Clinical manifestations and early diagnosis of Sjogren syndrome. *Archives of internal medicine.* 2004; 164(12): 1275-84.

[26] Fox RI, Liu AY. Sjogren's syndrome in dermatology. *Clinics in dermatology.* 2006; 24(5):393-413.

[27] Ramos-Casals M, Brito-Zeron P, Siso-Almirall A, Bosch X. Primary Sjogren syndrome. *Bmj.* 2012; 344:e3821.

[28] Fox RI. Sjögren's syndrome. *The Lancet.* 2005; 366(9482):321-31.

[29] Moerman RV, Bootsma H, Kroese FG, Vissink A. Sjogren's syndrome in older patients: aetiology, diagnosis and management. *Drugs & aging.* 2013; 30(3): 137-53.

[30] Tristano AG. The impact of rheumatic diseases on sexual function. *Rheumatology international.* 2009; 29(8):853-60.

[31] Marchesoni D, Mozzanega B, De Sandre P, Romagnolo C, Gambari PF, Maggino T. Gynaecological aspects of primary Sjogren's syndrome.

*European journal of obstetrics, gynecology, and reproductive biology.* 1995; 63(1):49-53.

[32] Skopouli FN, Dafni U, Ioannidis JP, Moutsopoulos HM. Clinical evolution, and morbidity and mortality of primary Sjogren's syndrome. *Seminars in arthritis and rheumatism.* 2000; 29(5): 296-304.

[33] Strimlan CV, Rosenow EC, 3rd, Divertie MB, Harrison EG, Jr. Pulmonary manifestations of Sjogren's syndrome. *Chest.* 1976; 70(03): 354-61.

[34] Garcia-Carrasco M, Ramos-Casals M, Rosas J, Pallares L, Calvo-Alen J, Cervera R, et al. Primary Sjogren syndrome: clinical and immunologic disease patterns in a cohort of 400 patients. *Medicine.* 2002; 81(4): 270-80.

[35] Mialon P, Barthelemy L, Sebert P, Le Henaff C, Sarni D, Pennec YL, et al. A longitudinal study of lung impairment in patients with primary Sjogren's syndrome. *Clinical and experimental rheumatology.* 1997; 15(4): 349-54.

[36] Ziza JM, Kaplan G, Salomon C, Kahn MF. [Severe pulmonary fibrosis disclosing primary Gougerot-Sjogren syndrome. Apropos of 5 cases, 2 of which were fatal]. *Annales de medecine interne.* 1986; 137(1):46-50.

[37] Ramos-Casals M, Font J, Garcia-Carrasco M, Brito MP, Rosas J, Calvo-Alen J, et al. Primary Sjogren syndrome: hematologic patterns of disease expression. *Medicine.* 2002; 81(4):281-92.

[38] Kyle Ra Fau - Gleich GJ, Gleich Gj Fau - Bayrid ED, Bayrid Ed Fau - Vaughan JH, Vaughan JH. *Benign hypergammaglobulinemic purpura of Waldenstrom.* (0025-7974 (Print)).

[39] Provost TT, Watson R, Simmons-O'Brien E. Anti-Ro(SS-A) antibody positive Sjogren's/lupus erythematosus overlap syndrome. *Lupus.* 1997; 6(2): 105-11.

[40] Konishi M, Ohosone Y, Matsumura M, Oyamada Y, Yamaguchi K, Kawahara Y, et al. Mixed-cryoglobulinemia associated with cutaneous vasculitis and pulmonary symptoms. *Internal medicine.* 1997; 36(1): 62-7.

[41] Ioannidis JP, Vassiliou VA, Moutsopoulos HM. Long-term risk of mortality and lymphoproliferative disease and predictive classification of primary Sjogren's syndrome. *Arthritis and rheumatism.* 2002; 46(3): 741-7.

[42] Pirildar T, Tikiz C, Ozkaya S, Tarhan S, Utuk O, Tikiz H, et al. Endothelial dysfunction in patients with primary Sjogren's syndrome. *Rheumatology international.* 2005; 25(7):536-9.

[43] Tektonidou M, Kaskani E, Skopouli FN, Moutsopoulos HM. Microvascular abnormalities in Sjogren's syndrome: nailfold capillaroscopy. *Rheumatology*. 1999; 38(9):826-30.

[44] Jubert C, Cosnes A, Clerici T, Gaulard P, Andre P, Revuz J, et al. Sjogren's syndrome and cutaneous B cell lymphoma revealed by anetoderma. *Arthritis and rheumatism*. 1993; 36(1):133-4.

[45] Belafsky PC, Postma GN. The laryngeal and esophageal manifestations of Sjogren's syndrome. *Current rheumatology reports*. 2003; 5(4): 297-303.

[46] Raderer M, Osterreicher C, Machold K, Formanek M, Fiebiger W, Penz M, et al. Impaired response of gastric MALT-lymphoma to Helicobacter pylori eradication in patients with autoimmune disease. *Annals of oncology : official journal of the European Society for Medical Oncology / ESMO*. 2001; 12(7):937-9.

[47] Collin P, Karvonen AL, Korpela M, Laippala P, Helin H. Gastritis classified in accordance with the Sydney system in patients with primary Sjogren's syndrome. *Scandinavian journal of gastroenterology*. 1997; 32(2): 108-11.

[48] Volter F, Fain O, Mathieu E, Thomas M. Esophageal function and Sjogren's syndrome. *Digestive diseases and sciences*. 2004; 49(2): 248-53.

[49] Tincani A, Andreoli L, Cavazzana I, Doria A, Favero M, Fenini MG, et al. Novel aspects of Sjogren's syndrome in 2012. *BMC medicine*. 2013; 11:93.

[50] Barendregt PJ, Visser MR, Smets EM, Tulen JH, van den Meiracker AH, Boomsma F, et al. Fatigue in primary Sjogren's syndrome. *Ann. Rheum. Dis*. 1998;57(5):291-5.

[51] Ng WF, Bowman SJ. Primary Sjogren's syndrome: too dry and too tired. *Rheumatology*. 2010;49(5):844-53.

[52] Segal B, Thomas W, Rogers T, Leon JM, Hughes P, Patel D, et al. Prevalence, severity, and predictors of fatigue in subjects with primary Sjogren's syndrome. *Arthritis and rheumatism*. 2008;59(12):1780-7.

[53] Goules AV, Tzioufas AG, Moutsopoulos HM. Classification criteria of Sjogren's syndrome. *Journal of autoimmunity*. 2014.

[54] Bossini N, Savoldi S, Franceschini F, Mombelloni S, Baronio M, Cavazzana I, et al. Clinical and morphological features of kidney involvement in primary Sjogren's syndrome. *Nephrology, dialysis, transplantation: official publication of the European Dialysis and*

*Transplant Association - European Renal Association.* 2001; 16(12): 2328-36.

[55] Kronbichler A, Mayer G. Renal involvement in autoimmune connective tissue diseases. *BMC medicine*. 2013;11:95.

[56] Ramos-Casals M, Tzioufas AG, Font J. Primary Sjogren's syndrome: new clinical and therapeutic concepts. *Ann. Rheum. Dis.* 2005; 64(3): 347-54.

[57] Lindvall B, Bengtsson A Fau - Ernerudh J, Ernerudh J Fau - Eriksson P, Eriksson P. *Subclinical myositis is common in primary Sjogren's syndrome and is not related to muscle pain.* (0315-162X (Print)).

[58] Ostuni P, Botsios C, Sfriso P, Bertagnin A, Cozzi F, Doria A, et al. [Prevalence and clinical features of fibromyalgia in systemic lupus erythematosus, systemic sclerosis and Sjogren's syndrome]. *Minerva medica.* 2002; 93(3):203-9.

[59] Fauchais AL, Magy L, Vidal E. Central and peripheral neurological complications of primary Sjogren's syndrome. *Presse medicale*. 2012; 41(9 Pt 2):e485-93.

[60] Delalande S, de Seze J, Fauchais AL, Hachulla E, Stojkovic T, Ferriby D, et al. Neurologic manifestations in primary Sjogren syndrome: a study of 82 patients. *Medicine.* 2004; 83(5):280-91.

[61] Mavragani CP, Fragoulis GE, Moutsopoulos HM. Endocrine alterations in primary Sjogren's syndrome: an overview. *Journal of autoimmunity.* 2012; 39(4):354-8.

[62] Fauchais AL, Ouattara B, Gondran G, Lalloue F, Petit D, Ly K, et al. Articular manifestations in primary Sjogren's syndrome: clinical significance and prognosis of 188 patients. *Rheumatology.* 2010; 49(6):1164-72.

[63] Voulgarelis M, Dafni UG, Isenberg DA, Moutsopoulos HM. Malignant lymphoma in primary Sjogren's syndrome: a multicenter, retrospective, clinical study by the European Concerted Action on Sjogren's Syndrome. *Arthritis and rheumatism.* 1999; 42(8):1765-72.

[64] Jonsson R, Moen K, Vestrheim D, Szodoray P. Current issues in Sjogren's syndrome. *Oral diseases.* 2002; 8(3):130-40.

[65] Solans-Laque R, Lopez-Hernandez A, Bosch-Gil JA, Palacios A, Campillo M, Vilardell-Tarres M. Risk, predictors, and clinical characteristics of lymphoma development in primary Sjogren's syndrome. *Seminars in arthritis and rheumatism.* 2011; 41(3):415-23.

[66] Kalk WW, Vissink A, Spijkervet FK, Bootsma H, Kallenberg CG, Nieuw Amerongen AV. Sialometry and sialochemistry: diagnostic tools

for Sjögren's syndrome. *Annals of the Rheumatic Diseases.* 2001; 60(12): 1110-6.

[67] Schall GL, Anderson LG, Wolf RO, Herdt JR, Tarpley TMJ, Cummings NA, et al. Xerostomia in Sjögren's syndrome. Evaluation by sequential salivary scintigraphy. *JAMA: The Journal Of The American Medical Association.* 1971; 216(13):2109-16.

[68] Lucca JA, Nunez JN, Farris RL. A comparison of diagnostic tests for keratoconjunctivitis sicca: lactoplate, Schirmer, and tear osmolarity. *The CLAO Journal: Official Publication Of The Contact Lens Association Of Ophthalmologists*, Inc. 1990; 16(2):109-12.

[69] Shiboski SC, Shiboski CH, Criswell LA, Baer AN, Challacombe S, Lanfranchi H, et al. American College of Rheumatology classification criteria for Sjögren's syndrome: A data-driven, expert consensus approach in the Sjögren's International Collaborative Clinical Alliance Cohort. *Arthritis Care & Research.* 2012; 64(4):475-87.

[70] Daniels TE. Salivary histopathology in diagnosis of Sjogren's syndrome. *Scandinavian journal of rheumatology Supplement.* 1986;61:36-43.

[71] Vitali C, Bombardieri S, Jonsson R, Moutsopoulos HM, Alexander EL, Carsons SE, et al. Classification criteria for Sjogren's syndrome: a revised version of the European criteria proposed by the American-European Consensus Group. *Annals of the Rheumatic Diseases.* 2002; 61(6):554-8.

[72] Vitali C, Bombardieri S, Moutsopoulos HM, Balestrieri G, Bencivelli W, Bernstein RM, et al. Preliminary criteria for the classification of Sjögren's syndrome. Results of a prospective concerted action supported by the European community. *Arthritis & Rheumatism.* 1993;36(3):340-7.

[73] Rasmussen A, Ice JA, Li H, Grundahl K, Kelly JA, Radfar L, et al. Comparison of the American-European Consensus Group Sjögren's syndrome classification criteria to newly proposed American College of Rheumatology criteria in a large, carefully characterised sicca cohort. *Annals of the Rheumatic Diseases.* 2014;73(1):31-8.

[74] Bowman SJ, Fox RI. Classification criteria for Sjogren's syndrome: nothing ever stands still! *Ann. Rheum. Dis.* 2014; 73(1):1-2.

*Reviewed by:* Germán Esparza-Gómez, Professor of Oral Medicine Faculty of Dentistry, Department of Medicine and Buccofacial Surgery, Complutense University of Madrid, Madrid, Spain. esparza@odon.ucm.es.

In: Sjögren's Syndrome
Editor: Eduardo M. Hernandez
ISBN: 978-1-63117-859-7


*Chapter IV*

# Health-Related Quality of Life and Sexual Health in Patients with Sjögren's Syndrome and with Not- Sjögren's Sicca Syndrome

***Angela Del Rosso**, *Susanna Maddali Bongi*†
*and Svetlana Mikhaylova*‡**
Department of Experimental and Clinical Medicine,
Division of Medicine, University of Florence, Italy

## Abstract

In primary Sjögren's Syndrome (pSS), health-related quality of life (HRQoL) and sexual health are impaired and correlated.

HRQoL in pSS is similarly altered in respect to patients with not Sjogren Sicca Syndrome (nS-SS) (presenting ocular and oral dryness, with negative autoantibodies and lip biopsy).

* Corresponding author: Angela Del Rosso, MD, PhD. Department of Experimental and Clinical Medicine, Division of Rheumatology, University of Florence. Viale Pieraccini, 18 – 50139 Florence, Telephone: +390554271022; e-mail angela.delrosso@fastwebnet.it.
† Susanna Maddali Bongi, MD, susanna.maddalibongi@gmail.com.
‡ Svetlana Mikhaylova, MD, svetlana.mkh@gmail.com.

As expected, in pSS and ns-SS, HRQoL is related to the involvement of salivary and lachrymal glands, causing mainly dryness. In pSS and nS-SS, HRQoL is associated with anxiety and fatigue and, only in pSS, with depression. Pain, muscle skeletal concerns, and lung involvement are other determinants of HRQoL in pSS.

In women with pSS and nS-SS, sex health and ability, similarly altered, are affected by gynecological concerns, such as vaginal and vulvar dryness, more than by muscle-skeletal symptoms and, importantly, are related to impaired HRQoL.

**Keywords:** Sjögren's Syndrome, not Sjogren Sicca Syndrome, health related quality of life, quality of life, sexual health, sexual disability, xerostomia, xerophalmia, vaginal dryness, vulvar dryness, fatigue, depression, anxiety.

*No financial supports or any other benefit which could create a potential conflict of interest with regard to the work are declared.*

## 1. Quality of Life, Health-Related Quality of Life and Sexual Health

*Quality of Life (Qol)* is defined by World Health Organization (WHO) as Individuals' perception of their position in life in the context of the culture and value systems in which they live and in relation to their goals, expectations, standards and concerns. It is a broad ranging concept affected in a complex way by the person's physical health, psychological state, level of independence, social relationships, personal beliefs and their relationship to salient features of their environment [1].

*Health-related quality of life (HRQoL)* is an individual's satisfaction or happiness with domains of life insofar as they affect or are affected by health. HRQoL can be distinguished from QoL in that it concerns itself primarily with those factors that fall under the purview of health care providers and health care systems [2].

Thus, assessment of HRQoL represents an attempt to determine how variables within the dimension of health (e.g., a disease or its treatment) relate to particular dimensions of life determined to be important to people in general (generic HRQoL) or to people who have a specific disease (condition-specific HRQoL). Most conceptualizations of HRQoL emphasize the effects of disease on physical and social role and on psychological, emotional, cognitive and sexual functioning [3].

HRQol is increasingly acknowledged as a valid, appropriate and significant indicator of service need and intervention outcomes in public health research and practice.

*Sexual health* is a state of physical, emotional, mental and social health in relation to sexuality, that is an integral part of self identity, body image and HRQoL [4].

## 2. Health-Related Quality of Life in Sjögren Syndrome and in Not-Sjögren's Sicca Syndrome

The wide range of symptoms of *Sjögren syndrome* (SS), derived from the involvement of exocrine glands and from extra glandular manifestations, could impair HRQoL. However, the importance of this aspect is under-evaluated in clinical practice and attention on the matter has been raised by specific studies only in the last 10 years.

In SS the main symptoms, xerostomia and xerophtalmia, are due to reduced secretion of salivary and lachrymal glands, but many different clinical manifestations, derived from the changes in other epithelia, including skin, urogenital, respiratory, and gastrointestinal tracts [5] may contribute to the discomfort of the patients.

HRQoL may be further impaired by extra glandular manifestations, referred in around 1/3 of In SS patients and represented by lung and renal disease, involvement of muscle skeletal system and nervous system, and small vessel vasculitis [6]. Moreover, fatigue, sometimes, severe, and psychological disorders, such as depression and anxiety, may be present since disease onset [7-8].

According to the American and European Consensus Group (AECG) classification criteria, *primary Sjögren syndrome (pSS)* is defined in the presence of any 4 of 6 listed criteria as long as either histopathology or serology (antibodies to Ro[SSA] and/or to La[SSB]) is positive [9].

Some works evaluating the influence of disease derived symptoms on HRQoL included also patients presenting ocular and salivary symptoms not fulfilling criteria for pSS, [9], considered as affected by *not-Sjögren sicca syndrome (nS-SS)* [10].

The wide array of symptoms renders pSS a complex disease, in which HRQoL is impaired when compared to general population [11-18] and to patients with Rheumatoid Arthritis [19].

In the different studies, HRQoL was assessed by different questionnaires, such as Short Form 36, (SF36), its concise versions Short Form 12 (SF 12) and Short Form 8 (SF 8), and by EuroQol-D5 and WHO-QoL-BREF.

The SF36 consists of 36 items organized into 8 domains measuring 8 health concepts: physical functioning (PF), role limitations due to physical problems (PP), bodily pain (BP), general health perceptions (GH), vitality (V), social functioning (SF), role limitations due to emotional problems (EP), and general mental health (MH), combined into a summary physical composite score (PCS) ) and a summary mental composite score (MCS), with higher scores corresponding to better HRQoL (range 0-100) [20]. The **SF12** is a 12-item subset of the SF-36, that measures the same 8 domains, combined into SPI and SMI, as reliable as SF36 in assessing HRQoL. Consistently with SF36, higher scores correspond to better HRQoL (range 0-100) [21].

The SF8 measures, by a single item for domain, the same 8 domains of SF36, combined into SPI and SMI. As in SF36, higher scores mean better HRQoL (range 0-100) [22].

The EuroQoL-D5 consists of 5 dimensions (mobility, self-care, usual activities, pain/discomfort and anxiety/depression) each of which can take one of 3 responses: no problems=1; some problems=2, extreme problems=3, generating a total of 243 possible health states, and a vertical 0-100 visual analogue scale (VAS), with the best imaginable health state = 100 and the worst imaginable health state = 0, respectively [23].

The WHOQoL-BREF, derived from WHOQoL-100 instrument, comprises 26 items grouped in 4 health areas (physical health, psychological health, social relationships, and environment) and 2 items measuring overall QoL and general health, with high scores indicating better QoL (range 0-100) [24].

Interestingly, most of the studies assessing HRQol in pSS and nS-SS did not show differences in HRQol between these groups, despite the different criteria used in the enrollment of nS-SS patients. Some studies compared HRQol of pSS patients with those not fulfilling AECG-criteria [25,12], other with patients reporting only xerostomia [26]. Champey et al. [27] enrolled sicca patients with asthenia or limb pain, without any autoimmune feature and Cho et al. [16] evaluated heterogeneous non-SS sicca subjects, including patients with dry eyes and mouth syndrome, dry eye syndrome, drug induced sicca, undifferentiated connective tissue disease and burning mouth syndrome.

Only one study [12] found significantly lower HRQol scores in pSS than in nS-SS patients, but sample size was relatively small (33 and 19 subjects, respectively) and almost half of the cases with pSS had an associated fibromyalgia syndrome, which also may impair HRQol.

The similar impact of HRQol in pSS and non-SS sicca patients is not a surprising finding, since these two populations reported similar clinical features [12,16,25-27]. These data are in agreement with a proposal made by some authors, who, due to high specificity and low sensitivity of AEGC criteria [9], considered patients fulfilling them and those presenting only with sicca symptoms and signs, as affected by the same condition, yielding a different disease expression [10,28]. For this reason, it was proposed to consider patients fulfilling AECG-criteria as affected by Sjögren disease and those with negative antibodies and biopsy as affected by Sjögren syndrome [10].

Although pSS and non-SS sicca patients reported comparable clinical features and similarly impaired HRQoL, its determinants were different between the two populations for what concerns ocular and oral manifestations, central derived symptoms, involvement of muscle-skeletal system and internal organs.

## 2.1. HRQoL in pSS and in nS-SS: Correlation with Ocular and Oral Manifestations

PSS patients, due to involvement of salivary and lachrymal glands [29], develop many oral and ocular symptoms including xerostomia, difficulty in eating, sandy filling, burning sensation and pain in the eyes, difficulty in reading, in watching a computer or a television screen [30,31]. These manifestations and complications such as fungal infections, oral ulcerations, and dental decay, [32] may induce severe psychological and social problems and may affect HRQol [33].

The symptoms and signs related to *ocular manifestations* are pivotal aspects for pSS and n-SS patients since their early onset. However, it was demonstrated that impaired HRQol is more closely related with subjective ocular dryness than with objective examination findings.

Mizuno et al. [25], found no significant correlation in pSS patients between any ocular surface examination finding (Schirmer test, fluorescein and rose Bengal staining scores) and SF8 subscales. Champay et al. [27], by bivariate analysis, showed that subjective ocular dryness (assessed by VAS) and Schirmer test were significantly related in pSS patients but not in patients with nS-SS. In spite of a high proportion of abnormal Schirmer scores, in patients with pSS, subjective ocular dryness and HRQoL were not significantly correlated. Conversely, in nS-SS patients, whose Schirmer test scores were similar to the normal range, subjective ocular dryness significantly affected MCS of SF36. These data show a discrepancy between objective examination findings and subjective severity reported by patients, especially in nS-SS group.

As regards *oral symptoms,* xerostomia, when assessed by VAS scores for oral dryness, seems not to be the most disturbing symptom for pSS and nS-SS patients [27]. In contrast, studies that used specific self-assessed questionnaires, reported significant impact of oral health on HRQol in pSS and nS-SS. Palm et al. [34] showed significant differences in five out of the eight SF36 subscales (physical role limitation, general health, social functioning, emotional role limitations, mental health) between the groups with high and low oral distress, evaluated by oral health impact profile 14 questionnaire (OHIP-14).

Accordingly, Stewart et al. [35] showed that OHIP-14 summary score correlated significantly, by multivariate analysis, with general health and social functioning subscales of SF-36. In the study of Cho et al. [16] the Xerostomia Inventory (XI) score (a tool assessing xerostomia by 11 items, whose responses were summated to give a single value [36]), was the main determinant of SF36 PCS in nS-SS patients.

Thus, the use of questionnaires specifically assessing the impact of oral health is recommended in both populations to evaluate the contribution of oral symptoms to impaired HRQol.

With this purpose, in future studies assessing determinants of HRQoL in pSS and ns-SS, it could be useful the inclusion of more recent validated questionnaires assessing the severity of sicca symptoms such as Sicca Symptoms Inventory (SSI) [37].

## 2.2. HRQoL in pSS and in nS-SS: Correlation with Central Derived Symptoms

Despite the high prevalence of mood disorders in pSS [17,19], the studies assessing their impact on HRQol in pSS, probably due to the use of different instruments and different cut-off values to define depression and anxiety, reported not homogeneous results.

In the study of Segal et al. [17] *depression*, evaluated by Center for Epidemiologic Studies Depression Scale (CESD), was present in 37% of pSS patients and was the main predictor of emotional role limitations subscale of SF36, accounting for 25% of its variance at multivariate analysis. Cho et al. [16] showed by multivariate analysis that depression was the main determinant of MCS in pSS; although its contribution to MCS variance was not reported. According to Lendrem et al. [13] depression, assessed by HADS-D (cut-off ≥5 in HADS-D subscale), was identified as one of the most important predictors of HRQol evaluated by EuroQol-D5, together with pain, accounting for 48% of its variability. Inal et al. [15] reported a prevalence of depression (based on a cut-off ≥7 in HADS-D subscale) of 31.1% in pSS, and lower scores in 3 out of 4 domains of WHOQoL-BREF in patients with depression than in those not depressed.

Few studies assessed the impact of *anxiety* on HRQol in pSS and nS-SS. In Inal study, its prevalence (based on a cut-off ≥ 10 in HADS-A subscale) was 30%. Anxious patients reported significantly lower scores in all WHOQoL-BREF subscales than those without anxiety, but HADS-A scores were not related with any of SF36 subscales [15]. In another study, anxiety (assessed by HADS-A) was a weak predictor of HRQol, together with fatigue and body mass index, accounting for only <5% of variance in EuroQol-D5 [13].

The limited data published on nS-SS patients indicate that HRQol may be more strongly affected by anxiety than by depression. Cho et al. [16] found that anxiety (evaluated by VAS) was the main determinant of MCS in nS-SS. From these data, it can be hypothesized that nS-SS patients, not reaching sufficient criteria to confirm SS diagnosis, although presenting the same subjective symptoms, can be more anxious about their future and disease progression than patients with an established diagnosis.

Studies in many populations reported that depression and anxiety are frequently comorbid conditions, that anxiety is primary to depression in the majority of comorbid cases, and that patients with anxiety are at higher risk to develop major depression [38,39]. Depressive patients with comorbid anxiety have a more difficult course and a decreased or a delayed response to treatment [40]. Thus, in pSS and nS-SS, an earlier identification of depression and anxiety and a determination of their contributing factors may be important to manage them and to improve HRQol of the patients.

*Fatigue* is ranked as one of the most disturbing symptoms in pSS [11,13]. However, studies assessing its contribution to HRQoL reported contradictory results.

In the study of Inal et al. [15], at multivariate regression analysis, fatigue, evaluated by VAS, was not independently associated of with any of SF36 subscales, while accounted, together with arthritis, for 35% and 31% of the variance in physical health and social relationship domains of WHOQoL-BREF, respectively.

Differently, according to Lendrem et al. [13] fatigue, assessed by Profile of Fatigue and Discomfort (Pro-F), was a relatively weak predictor of EuroQoL-5D, accounting only for 2% of its variance. Somatic fatigue, assessed by Profile of Fatigue and Discomfort-Sicca Symptoms Inventory (PROFAD-SSI) contributed to 7% and 8% of the variance of SF36 physical function and general health scales, respectively, in the study by Segal et al. [17].

Meijer et al. [11] showed that presence of fatigue was independently associated with reduced scores of MCS and PCS of SF36, although contribution of fatigue to their scores was not reported. Ibn Yacoub et al. [41] reported a significant association of all MAF (Multidimensional assessment of fatigue) and SF-36 domains in bivariate analysis.

In the only study evaluating nS-SS patients, fatigue, assessed by VAS, correlated in bivariate analysis with SMI and SMI score in with nS-SS and only with PCS in pSS, and was similar in the two populations [27].

Although fatigue is the one of most disturbing symptom for pSS and nS-SS patients, the mechanisms by which it may impair HRQol are not clear. There are contrasting data about the correlation of fatigue levels with disease activity markers in pSS. Fatigue was related with anti-SSB antibodies [42], with the total level of immunoglobulins and trombocyte counts [43], but other works did not show correlation of fatigue with serum cytokine levels [44][26], nor with anti-SSA and anti-SSB antibodies and immunoglobulins G [45].

The similar levels of fatigue in ns-SS [27], may lead to hypothesize that inflammatory and auto-immune features do not contribute significantly to fatigue in pSS patients.

It is known that psychological variables (*mainly* depression) are strong determinants of fatigue in pSS, [43,46,47]. Although fatigue was reported by depressive patients, it was also experienced in the absence of depression, suggesting that these features may be independent but interrelated [46]. Thus, in pSS patients, HRQoL may be affected indirectly by fatigue due, on its part, to depressive symptoms or, independently, by both of them.

Paying tribute to the huge importance of fatigue in pSS and nS-SS patients, it is advisable to assess its presence not only by a single question, but by specific validated questionnaires, in order to better characterize severity of fatigue and to detect its improvement in response to therapeutic interventions.

## 2.3. HRQoL in pSS and in nS-SS: Correlation with Muscle-Skeletal Symptoms and Pain

*Muscle-skeletal manifestations* occur in approximately 30-60% of patients with pSS [48]. Interestingly, symptoms of joints and muscles involvement affect physical as well as mental domains of SF36. Mejer et al. [11] showed by multivariate analysis that tendomyalgia and arthralgia in pSS patients were associated with PCS and MCS, respectively. Accordingly, Inal et al. [15] found that physical function, physical role limitation, emotional role difficulties, social functioning and mental health subscales of SF36 were associated with arthralgia. The number of swollen and tender joints was significantly associated with all subscales of SF36, except than with physical functioning [41], while pain was an independent predictor of SF36 emotional problems and physical functioning [17].

The only study assessing impact of muscle-skeletal symptoms on HRQol in nS-SS patients reported association of joint or muscle pain with PCS of SF36 in both pSS and nS-SS populations [27].

Since none of these studies assessed the association of arthralgia and tendomyalgia with inflammatory parameters, it is not clear if these symptoms may be caused by pathological process in muscle skeletal system or have another origin. Interestingly, in different studies, from 18% to 50% of pSS patients reported an associated *fibromyalgia* syndrome [49-51]. Thus, pSS and nS-SS patients reporting muscle-skeletal pain should be evaluated for the presence of fibromyalgia symptoms to better understand the mechanisms of pain and its influence on HRQoL, thus to properly target pain management and to improve HRQol.

## 2.4. HRQoL in pSS and in nS-SS: Correlation with Internal Organs Manifestations

Among internal organ manifestations, lung involvement results the most important predictors of HRQol in pSS.

In the study of Palm et al. [52], pSS patients with lung involvement (defined as pulmonary symptoms and either abnormal findings on high resolution computerized tomography, or pulmonary function tests ≤75% of predicted values) presented significantly lower scores in SF36 physical functioning score than those without lung involvement. Stewart et al. [35] showed that self reported symptoms of renal, cardiovascular, pulmonary and gastrointestinal involvement were significantly correlated to all eight SF 36 domains. Thus, in pSS patients with impaired HRQol, potential extra glandular manifestations, especially lung involvement, should be ruled out.

### 2.5. HRQol in pSS: Correlation with Indexes of Disease Damage or Activity

In pSS, *Disease Damage Index* (DDI) (assessing oral/salivary, ocular, neurological, pleuropulmonary damages, renal impairment and lymphoproliferative disease, weighed from 1 to 5) [53] was significantly and negatively correlated with the general health score of SF36 [35].

Accordingly, *EULAR Sjögren's syndrome patients reported index* (ESSPRI), calculating the weights of the each domain and the mean final score [54], was a significant independent predictor of SF36 PCS score [16].

The use of specific indexes, calculated by the sum of the several domains, as potential predictors of impaired HRQol in pSS patients is disputable. Since they do not provide information about single domains, it is difficult to evaluate which of their domains may impact HRQoL and, thus, to individuate interventions to improve HRQol. Arguably, in the assessment of pSS patients, the inclusion of instruments reporting also the weights of the each domain, such as ESSPRI, may be helpful. However, longitudinal studies, evaluating whether any of above-mentioned indexes could be associated with changes in HRQol scores over time, are needed.

## 3. Sexual Health in Patients with Sjögren Syndrome and with Not-Sjögren Sicca Syndrome

Sexual health is linked with health status and is an important part of HRQoL because the psychological and physical changes occurring in patients suffering from chronic diseases may lead to changes in perceived HRQoL and quality of sexual life and to impairment in sexual functioning.

Sexual functioning, consisting in sexual activity with transition through the phases from arousal to relaxation and with a feeling of pleasure, fulfillment and satisfaction [55, 56] is impaired in chronic systemic rheumatic diseases such as Rheumatoid Arthritis [57,58], Ankylosing Spondylitis [59], Systemic Lupus Erythematosus [60], and Systemic Sclerosis [61] due to physical and psychological factors, potentially reducing sexual desire, satisfaction and frequency of intercourses [62].

However, in rheumatic diseases, sexual health and functioning are under evaluated in daily practice and seldom included in clinical studies. Moreover, items assessing sex are included only in two questionnaires (WHO disability assessment schedule II -WHO-DAS II- and International Classification of Functioning –ICF- core sets for Rheumatoid Arthritis) [63,64] and instruments specifically evaluating sexual function are rarely used.

Due to the involvement of genital tract epithelia and glands, in women with pSS, *gynecological concerns*, such as vulvar and vaginal dryness [65-69], dyspareunia [70-72], pruritus, genital pain, increased susceptibility to infection and dysuria are frequent in the course of the disease and may potentially precede by many years the onset of ocular or oral symptoms [69-71].

Although in literature a high prevalence of gynecological symptoms in pSS is reported, there are scanty data on their impact on sexual ability and activity.

Our group found that, both in women with pSS and with nS-SS, *sex disability affected HRQoL* (evaluated by SF36), other than global disability, mood and fatigue. Lower scores in PCS were shown in patients with pSS not having a sexual relationship, in those not feeling pleasure during sexual activity and in nS-SS patients with dysuria, who also presented lower SF36 MCS scores [73].

At the best of our knowledge, our study was the only work assessing gynecological symptoms and sex disability in women with nS-SS versus pSS. By a modified version of Hill Questionnaire [74] evaluating the impact of nS-SS and pSS on sexual activity, relationship with the partner, and communication about sex issues by 16 questions, we showed a high prevalence both of gynecological symptoms (especially vulvar and vaginal dryness) and sex disability, resulting similar in the two populations.

Gynecological concerns, more than muscle-skeletal symptoms, altered sex activity both in nS-SS and pSS. All the aspects related to sexual behavior, such as sexual relationship with the partner, frequency of intercourses, sexual drive, pleasure and satisfaction, were severely impaired by the disease similarly in the two groups.

Our results were partially different from a previous work showing no differences in women with pSS in respect to healthy controls in sexual activity (intended as intercourse frequency), libido and satisfaction (evaluated by single questions) although women with pSS presented a higher prevalence of dyspareunia and vaginal dryness than controls. Moreover, in pSS, differently from controls, the intercourse frequency did not diminish with age, nor was related with dyspareunia and disease duration [75].

The influence of circulating levels of androgens on sexual life, assessed by the McCoy scale (evaluating by 10 sub-scales frequency of intercourse, orgasm frequency, sexual pleasure and satisfaction, lubrication, dyspareunia, arousal, sexual fantasies, and satisfaction with partner) was evaluated by Valtysdottir et al. They found significant correlations of reduced dehydroepiandrosterone sulphate serum levels with the total McCoy score, as well with its subscales reflecting arousal, desire, and satisfaction. Thus, the authors propose the restoration of DHEA-S to normal circulating levels as a possible treatment to improve the quality of sexual life [76].

For women affected with pSS and ns-SS, the *communication* with the partner and with health care providers about the symptoms related to genital involvement and sex ability altered by their underlying diseases may be problematic. Interestingly, in our study, we found that the majority of patients had discussed about their health with the partners, who, in most cases, were sensitive to difficulties caused by the disease, allowing not to put a strain on the relationship. Differently, few patients were asked by health care providers if their disease had affected sexuality, and few of them approached someone else to discuss about sex problems [73].

These data are in agreement with previous results obtained in a group of women with SSc, 1/3 of whom suffered from a concomitant Sjögren's Syndrome. In this study, among the patients who answered to a specific questionnaire, only 60% of them had discussed sexual issues with health care providers, who focused more on other gynecologic issues rather than on sexual response [77].

These results highlight the reciprocal lack of communication about disease-related gynecological and sexual problems between health care providers and women with pSS and nS-SS, and indicate that health care providers need to be aware of these concerns, to help women to discuss them, and to seek solutions in order, ultimately, to improve patients well being and HRQoL.

# Conclusion

In pSS and nS-SS, the impairment of HRQoL is frequent, similar in the two conditions and related to disease manifestations due to the involvement of salivary and lachrymal glands and to the changes in other epithelial tissues. Also fatigue, anxiety, depression and extra-glandular manifestations, such as muscle skeletal concerns and lung involvement, may contribute to HRQoL impairment.

In women with pSS and nS-SS, sexual health and ability are similarly altered and, importantly, are related to impaired HRQoL. Sex ability is affected more by gynecological concerns, due to the involvement of glands of external genital tract, than by muscle-skeletal symptoms.

Both HRQoL and sexual health are rarely assessed and under-evaluated by health care providers in the management of patients with pSS and nS-SS.

Thus, the communication between patient and doctors about these themes is not sufficient and should be improved. In pSS and nS-SS, HRQoL and sexual health should be taken into account, assessed routinely with specific tests and questionnaires by rheumatologists and health professionals in the clinical practice, and treated with a multidisciplinary approach in collaboration with specialists such as psychologists and gynecologists. Moreover, longitudinal studies are advocated to investigate whether any clinical, clinimetric or laboratory variables at baseline could be associated with changes in HRQoL or sexual health in pSS and nS-SS over time.

# References

[1] WHOQOL Group. Development of the WHOQOL: Rationale and current status. *Int J. Mental Health* 1994; 23: 24–56.

[2] Wilson IB, Cleary PD. Linking clinical variables with health-related quality of life. *JAMA* 1995;1995:59-65.

[3] Ware JE. The status of health assessment 1994. *An Rev Pub Health* 1995;16:327-354.

[4] http://www.who.int/topics/sexual_health/en/ (accessed 18th February 2014).

[5] Fox RI. Sjögren's Syndrome. *Lancet.* 2005;366:321–31.

[6] Tzioufas AG, Vlachoyiannopoulos PG. Sjögren's Syndrome: an update on clinical, basic and diagnostic therapeutic aspects. *J. Autoimmun* 2012;39:1-3.

[7] Peri Y, Agmon-Levin N, Theodor E, Shoenfeld Y. Sjögren's syndrome, the old and the new. *Best Pract Res Clin. Rheumatol.* 2012;26:105-17.

[8] Morreale M, Marchione P, Giacomini P, Pontecorvo S, Marianetti M, Vento C, Tinelli E, Francia A. Neurological involvement in primary Sjögren syndrome: a focus on central nervous system. *PLoS One*. 2014 20;9:e84605.

[9] Vitali C, Bombardieri S, Jonsson R, Moutsopoulos HM, Alexander EL, Carsons SE, Daniels TE, Fox PC, Fox RI, Kassan SS, Pillemer SR, Talal N, Weisman MH; European Study Group on Classification Criteria for Sjögren's Syndrome: Classification criteria for Sjögren's syndrome: a revised version of the European criteria proposed by the American-European Consensus Group. *Ann. Rheum Dis* 2002; 61: 554-8.

[10] Ramos-Casals M, Brito-Zerón P, Perez-De-Lis M, Jimenez I, Blanco MJ, Bove A, Soto MJ, Akasbi M, Diaz C, Sentís J, Siso A. Sjögren syndrome or Sjögren disease? The histological and immunological bias caused by the 2002 criteria. *Clin. Rev. Allergy Immunol* 2010; 38: 178-5.

[11] Meijer JM, Meiners PM, James JR, Huddleston Slater JJ, Spijkervet FK, Kallenberg CG, Vissink A, Bootsma. Health-related quality of life, employment and disability in patients with Sjögren's syndrome. Rheumatology (Oxford) 2009;48:1077–82.

[12] Lopez-Jornet P, Camacho-Alonso F. Quality of life in patients with Sjögren's syndrome and sicca complex. *Journal of Oral Rehabilitation* 2008 35; 875–81.

[13] Lendrem D, Mitchell S, McMeekin P, Bowman S, Price E, Pease CT, Emery P, Andrews J, Lanyon P, Hunter J, Gupta M, Bombardieri M, Sutcliffe N, Pitzalis C, McLaren J, Cooper A, Regan M, Giles I, Isenberg D, Vadivelu S, Coady D, Dasgupta B, McHugh N, Young-Min S, Moots R, Gendi N, Akil M, Griffiths B, Ng WF; on behalf of the UK primary Sjögren's Syndrome Registry. Health-related utility values of patients with primary Sjögren's syndrome and its predictors. *Ann Rheum. Dis* 2013 Jun 12 [Epub ahead of print]doi:10.1136/annrheumdis-2012-202863.

[14] Kamel UF, Maddison P, Whitaker R. Impact of primary Sjögren's syndrome on smell and taste: effect on quality of life. *Rheumatology* (Oxford) 2009;48:1512–14.

[15] Inal V, Kitapcioglu G, Karabulut G, Keser G, Kabasakal Y. Evaluation of quality of life in relation to anxiety and depression in primary Sjo¨gren's syndrome. *Mod. Rheumatol* 2010; 20:588–97.

[16] Cho HJ, Yoo JJ, Yun CY, Kang EH, Lee HJ, Hyon JY, Song YW, Lee YJ. The EULAR Sjögren's syndrome patient reported index as an independent determinant of health-related quality of life in primary Sjögren's syndrome patients: in comparison with non-Sjögren's sicca patients. *Rheumatology* (Oxford). 2013;52:2208-17.

[17] Segal B, Bowman SJ, Philip C Fox PC, Vivino FB, Murukutla N, Brodscholl J, Ogale S, McLean L. Primary Sjögren's Syndrome: health experiences and predictors of health quality among patients in the United States. *Health and Quality of Life Outcomes* 2009; 7:46. doi: 10.1186/1477-7525-7-46.

[18] Strömbeck B, Ekdahl C, Manthorpe R, Wikström I, Jacobsson LHealth-related quality of life in primary Sjögren's syndrome, rheumatoid arthritis and fibromyalgia compared to normal population data using SF-36. *Scand J. Rheumatol*. 2000;29:20-8.

[19] Valtýsdóttir ST, Gudbjörnsson B, Lindqvist U, Hällgren R, Hetta J. Anxiety and depression in patients with primary Sjögren's syndrome. *J. Rheumatol.* 2000;27:165-9.

[20] Apolone G, Cifani S, Liberati MC, Mosconi P. Questionario sullo stato di salute SF-36. Traduzione e validazione della versione italiana: risultati del progetto IQOLA [Italian]. SF-36 questionnaire. Translation and validation of the Italian version. Metodologia e Didattica Clinica 1997;5:86-94.

[21] Ware J Jr, Kosinski M, Keller SD. A 12-Item Short-Form Health Survey: construction of scales and preliminary tests of reliability and validity. *Med Care* 1996; 34:220-33.

[22] Ware JE, Kosinski M, Dewey JE, Gandek B. How to Score and Interpret Single-Item Health Status Measures: A Manual for Users of the SF-8 Health Survey. Lincoln RI: QualityMetric Incorporated, 2001.

[23] Dolan P. Modeling valuations for EuroQol health states. *Med Care* 1997; 35:1095-108.

[24] Skevington SM, Lotfy M, O'Connell KA; WHOQOL Group. The World Health Organization's WHOQOL-BREF quality of life assessment: psychometric properties and results of the international field trial. A report from the WHOQOL group. *Qual Life Res.* 2004;13:299-310.

[25] Mizuno Y, Yamada M, Miyake Y. Association Between Clinical Diagnostic Tests and Health-Related Quality of Life Surveys in Patients with Dry Eye Syndrome. *Jpn J Ophthalmol* 2010;54:259–65.

[26] Rostron J, Rogers S, Longman L, Kancy S, Field EA. Health-related quality of life in patients with Primary Sjögren's Syndrome and Xerostomia: a comparative study. *Gerodontology*. 2002;19:53-9.

[27] Champey J, Corruble E, Gottenberg JE, Buhl C, Meyer T, Caudmont C et al. Quality of Life and Psychological Status in Patients With Primary Sjögren's Syndrome and Sicca Symptoms Without Autoimmune Features. *Arthritis Rheum* 2006; 55,3:451-7.

[28] Baldini C, Talarico R, Tzioufas AG, Bombardieri S. Classification criteria for Sjögren's Syndrome: a critical review. *J. Autoimmun.* 2012;39:9-14.

[29] Delaleu N, Jonsson MV, Appel S, Jonsson R. New concepts in the pathogenesis of Sjögren's syndrome. *Rheum. Dis. Clin North Am* 2008; 34: 833–45.

[30] Rehman HU. Sjögren syndrome. Yonsei Med J. 2003 30;44:947-54.

[31] Miljanovic B, Dana R, Sullivan DA, Schaumberg DA. Impact of dry eye syndrome on vision-related quality of life. *Am. J. Ophthalmol* 2007;143:409–15.

[32] Soto-Rojas AE, Kraus A. The oral side of Sjögren syndrome. Diagnosis and treatment. A review. *Arch Med Res* 2002; 33:95–106.

[33] Reisine ST, Fertig J, Weber J, Leder S. Impact of dental conditions on patient's quality of life. *Community Dent Oral Epidemiol* 1989; 17: 7–10.

[34] Enger TB, Palm Ø, Garen T, Sandvik L, Jensen JL. Oral distress in primary Sjögren syndrome: implications for health-related quality of life. *Eur. J. Oral Sci.* 2011; 119: 474–80.

[35] Stewart CM, Berg KM, Cha S and Reeves WH. Connection Sjögren Syndrome: A critical oral-systemic connection. *JADA* 2008;139:291-99.

[36] Thomson WM, Chalmers JM, Spencer AJ, Williams SM. The Xerostomia Inventory: a multi-item approach to measuring dry mouth. *Community Dent Health.* 1999;16:12-7.

[37] Bowman SJ, Booth DA, Platts RG, Field A, Rostron J; UK Sjögren's Interest Group. Validation of the Sicca Symptoms Inventory for clinical studies of Sjögren's syndrome. *J. Rheumatol.* 2003;30:1259-66.

[38] Sartorius N, Ustun TB, Lecrubier Y, Wittchen HU. Depression comorbid with anxiety: results from the WHO study on psychological

disorders in primary health care. *Br. J. Psychiatry* 1996;(Suppl 30):38-43.

[39] Wittchen HU, Kessler RC, Pfister H, Lieb M. Why do people with anxiety disorders become depressed? A prospective-longitudinal community study. *Acta Psychiatr Scand* 2000; 102 Suppl 406:14–23.18.

[40] Gum AM, Cheavens JS. Psychiatric comorbidity and depression in older adults. *Curr Psychiatry Rep*. 2008;10:23-9.

[41] Ibn Yacoub Y, Rostom S, Laatiris A, Hajjaj-Hassouni N. Primary Sjögren's syndrome in Moroccan patients: characteristics, fatigue and quality of life. *Rheumatol Int* 2012; 32:2637–43.

[42] Hansen B, Manthorpe R. Antibodies against SS-B/La and SS-A/Ro antigens in patients with primary Sjögren's syndrome. *Scand J Rheumatol* 1986;61:93–7.

[43] Bax HI, Vriesendorp TM, Kallenberg CG, Kalk WW. Fatigue and immune activity in Sjögren's syndrome. *Ann Rheum Dis* 2002;61:284.

[44] Hartkamp A, Geenen R, Bijl M, Kruize AA, Godaert GL, Derksen RH. Serum cytokine levels related to multiple dimensions of fatigue in patients with primary Sjögren's syndrome. *Ann. Rheum Dis* 2004, 63:1335-7.

[45] Haldorsen K, Bjelland I, Bolstad AI, Jonsson R, Brun JG. A five-year prospective study of fatigue in primary Sjögren's syndrome. *Arthritis Res Ther* 2011, 13:R167.

[46] Segal B, Thomas W, Rogers T, Leon JM, Hughes P, Patel D, Patel K, Novitzke J, Rohrer M, Gopalakrishnan R, Myers S, Nazmul-Hossain A, Emamian E, Huang A, Rhodus N, Moser K: Prevalence, severity, and predictors of fatigue in Primary Sjögren's Syndrome. Arthritis Rheum. 2008 15; 59: 1780–7.

[47] Barendregt PJ, Visser MR, Smets EM, Tulen JH, van den Meiracker AH, Boomsma F, Markusse HM: Fatigue in primary Sjögren's syndrome. *Ann Rheum Dis* 1998, 57:291-5.

[48] Fauchais AL, Ouattara B, Gondran G, Lalloué F, Petit D, Ly K, Lambert M, Launay D, Loustaud-Ratti V, Bezanahari H, Liozon E, Hachulla E, Jauberteau MO, Vidal E, Hatron PY. Articular manifestations in primary Sjögren's syndrome: clinical significance and prognosis of 188 patients. *Rheumatology* (Oxford). 2010;49:1164-72.

[49] Iannuccelli C, Spinelli FR, Guzzo MP, Priori R, Conti F, Ceccarelli F, Pietropaolo M, Olivieri M, Minniti A, Alessandri C, Gattamelata A, Valesini G, Di Franco M. Fatigue and widespread pain in systemic lupus erythematosus and Sjögren's syndrome: symptoms of the inflammatory

disease or associated fibromyalgia? *Clin Exp Rheumatol*. 2012;30: S117-21.

[50] Dohrenbusch R, Grüterich M, Genth E. Fibromyalgia and Sjögren syndrome--clinical and methodological aspects. [Article in German] Z *Rheumatol*. 1996;55:19-27.

[51] Vitali C, Tavoni A, Neri R, Castrogiovanni P, Pasero G, Bombardieri S. Fibromyalgia features in patients with primary Sjögren's syndrome. Evidence of a relationship with psychological depression. *Scand J Rheumatol* 1989; 18:21-27.

[52] Palm O, Garen T, Berge Enger T, Jensen JL, Lund MB, Aaløkken TM, Gran JT. Clinical pulmonary involvement in primary Sjögren's syndrome: prevalence, quality of life and mortality-a retrospective study based on registry data. *Rheumatology* 2013;52:173-9.

[53] Vitali C, Palombi G, Baldini C, Benucci M, Bombardieri S, Covelli M, Del Papa N, De Vita S, Epis O, Franceschini F, Gerli R, Govoni M, Bongi SM, Maglione W, Migliaresi S, Montecucco C, Orefice M, Priori R, Tavoni A, Valesini G. Sjögren's Syndrome Disease Damage Index and disease activity index: scoring systems for the assessment of disease damage and disease activity in Sjögren's syndrome, derived from an analysis of a cohort of Italian patients. *Arthritis Rheum* 2007;56:2223-31.

[54] Seror R, Ravaud P, Mariette X, Bootsma H, Theander E, Hansen A, Ramos-Casals M, Dörner T, Bombardieri S, Hachulla E, Brun JG, Kruize AA, Praprotnik S, Tomsic M, Gottenberg JE, Devauchelle V, Devita S, Vollenweider C, Mandl T, Tzioufas A, Carsons S, Saraux A, Sutcliffe N, Vitali C, Bowman SJ; EULAR Sjögren's Task Force. EULAR Sjögren's Syndrome patient reported index (ESSPRI): development of a consensus patient index for primary Sjögren's Syndrome. *Ann Rheum Dis* 2011;70: 968-72.

[55] Prady J, Vale A, Hill J. Body image and sexuality. In: Hill J (ed) Rheumatology nursing: a creative approach. Churchill Livingstone, Edinburgh, pp 109–124, 1998.

[56] Wells D. Caring for sexuality in health and illness. Churchill Livingstone, Edinburgh, 2000.

[57] Hill J, Bird H, Thorpe R. Effects of rheumatoid arthritis on sexual activity and relationships. *Rheumatology* (Oxford) 2003;42:280–6.

[58] Gossec L, Solano C, Paternotte S, Beauvais C, Gaudin P, von Krause G, Sordet C, Perdriger A. Elaboration and validation of a questionnaire

(Qualisex) to assess the impact of rheumatoid arthritis on sexuality with patient involvement. *Clin. Exp. Rheumatol* 2012;30:505-13.

[59] Healey EL, Haywood KL, Jordan KP, Garratt AM, Ryan S, Packham JC. Ankylosing spondylitis and its impact on sexual relationships. *Rheumatology* 2009; 48:1378-1381.

[60] Curry SL, Levine SB, Corty E, Jones PK, Kurit DM. The impact of systemic lupus erythematosus on women's sexual functioning. *J. Rheumatol.* 1994; 21: 2254-60.

[61] Schouffoer AA, van der Marel J, Ter Kuile MM, Weijenborg PT, Voskuyl A, Vliet Vlieland CW, van Laar JM, Vliet Vlieland TP.. Impaired Sexual Function in Women With Systemic Sclerosis: A Cross-Sectional Study. *Arthritis Rheum* 2009; 61:1601-8.

[62] Ostensen M. New insights into sexual functioning and fertility in rheumatic diseases. *Best Pract Res Clin Rheumatol* 2004; 18: 219-32.

[63] Hudson M, Steele R, Taillefer S, Baron M; Canadian Scleroderma Research. Quality of life in systemic sclerosis: psychometric properties of the World Health Organization Disability Assessment Schedule II. *Arthritis Rheum*. 2008;59:270-8.

[64] Stucki G, Cieza A, Geyh S, Battistella L, Lloyd J, Symmons D, Kostanjsek N, Schouten J. ICF Core Sets for rheumatoid arthritis. *J Rehabil Med.* 2004;(44 Suppl):87-93.

[65] Block KJ, Buchanan WW, Wohl MJ, Burnim, JJ. Sjögren's Syndrome. A clinical, pathological and serological study in 62 cases. *Medicine* 1965; 44: 187-231.

[66] Capriello P, Barale E, Capelli N, Lupo S, Teti G. Sjögren's Syndrome: clinical, cytological, histological and colposcopic aspects in women. *Clin. Exp. Obst Gyn* 1988; 15: 9-12.

[67] Al-Hashimi I, Khuder S, Haghighat N, Zipp M. Frequency and predictive value of the clinical manifestations in Sjögren's Syndrome. *J. Oral Pathol Med.* 2001; 30:1-6.

[68] Marchesoni D, Mozzanega B, De Sandre P, Romagnolo C, Gambari PF, Maggino T. Gynaecological aspects of primary Sjögren's Syndrome. *European Journal of Obstetrics & Gynecology and Reproductive Biology* 1995; 63: 49-53.

[69] Lehrer S, Bogursky E, Yemini M, Kase NG, Birkenfeld A. Gynecologic manifestations of Sjögren's Syndrome. *American Journal of Obstetrics and Gynecology*, 1994; 17: 835-7.

[70] Sellier S, Courville P, Joly P. Dyspareunia and Sjögren's Syndrome. *Ann Dermatol Venereol.* 2006; 133:17-20.

[71] Mulherin DM, Sheeran TP, Kumararatne DS, Speculand B, Luesley D, Situnayake RD. Sjögren's syndrome in women presenting with chronic dyspareunia. *Br J Obstet Gynaecol.* 1997;104:1019-23.

[72] Latt AE, Zinner SH, McCormack WM. The prevalence of dyspareunia. *Obstet Gynecol* 1990: 75:433-6.

[73] Maddali Bongi S, Del Rosso A, Olandi M, Matucci-Cerinic M. Gynaecological symptoms and sexual disability in women with primary Sjögren's syndrome and sicca syndrome. *Clin Exp Rheumatol.* 2013;3:683-90.

[74] Hill J, Bird H, Thorpe R. Effects of rheumatoid arthritis on sexual activity and relationships. *Rheumatology* (Oxford) 2003; 42: 280-6.

[75] Skopouli FN, Papanikolaou S, Malamou-Mitsi V, Papanikolaou N, Moutsopoulos HM. Obstetric and gynaecological profile in patients with primary Sjögren's syndrome. *Ann Rheum Dis*. 1994;53:569-73.

[76] Valtysdottir ST, Wide L, Hallgren R. Mental wellbeing and quality of sexual life in women with primary Sjögren'ssyndrome are related to circulating dehydroepiandrosterone sulphate. *Ann. Rheum Dis.* 2003;62:875-9.

[77] Saad, SC, Pietrzykowski, JE., Lewis, SS., Stepien AM, Latham VA, Messick S, Ensz SL, Wetherell C, Behrendt AE. Vaginal lubrication in women with scleroderma and Sjögren's Syndrome. *Sexuality and Disability* 1999; 17, 103-113.

In: Sjögren's Syndrome
Editor: Eduardo M. Hernandez
ISBN: 978-1-63117-859-7


*Chapter V*

# Involvement of the Central Nervous System in Sjögren's Syndrome

***Sandra Gofinet Pasoto** M.D., Ph.D.***
***and Tamyris de Sousa Bocate***
Rheumatology Division, University of São Paulo, São Paulo, Brazil

## Abstract

Primary Sjögren's syndrome (pSS) (or Sjögren's syndrome) is a chronic autoimmune inflammatory disease characterized primarily by involvement of the exocrine glands. Multiple organs may also be affected, causing a highly variable spectrum of clinical manifestations. Most patients have less severe extraglandular symptoms such as fatigue, polyarthralgia and diffuse myalgia, while others develop serious systemic impairments including pneumonitis, vasculitis, peripheral neuropathy, glomerulonephritis and lymphoma. The disease predominantly affects females, with a peak incidence between 40-60 years-old, and its prevalence in the general population is approximately 0.1-0.5%. The etiology is unknown, but the autoimmune nature of SS is supported by the production of multiple circulating autoantibodies, mainly anti-Ro/SSA and anti-La/SSB. Peripheral nervous system (PNS) involvement

* Corresponding author: Sandra Gofinet Pasoto, e-mail: sandrapasoto@yahoo.com.br.

is a well-recognized injury in this disease, which affects 10-20% of pSS patients. It is characterized by peripheral symmetric axonal sensorimotor polyneuropathy or pure sensory neuropathy. Central nervous system (CNS) involvement in pSS, although uncommon (0.3-6%), may aggravate the patient's clinical condition and lead to motor and cognitive sequelae. Retrospective studies assessing CNS damage in pSS suggest that the neurological manifestations are highly heterogeneous. In the series of Delalande et al. (2004), consisting of 56 pSS patients with CNS disorders referred to a neurologic department, focal or multifocal manifestations of the brain and/or spinal cord territories (including multiple sclerosis-like disease) were observed in all patients, whereas diffuse brain injuries were rare. In contrast, Massara et al. (2010) found CNS disorders in 6% of 424 pSS patients followed at a rheumatology unit, with predominance of diffuse manifestations (40%), including psychosis. This discrepancy could be explained by specific aspects of each study center (i.e., patients recruited from departments of internal medicine or neurology), the characteristics of the cohorts evaluated and also the different definitions and methods used for the diagnosis of neurological complications (i.e., whether or not including asymptomatic patients). In this chapter, the frequency, pathogenesis, clinical features, diagnosis, differential diagnosis and treatment of the central nervous system involvement in pSS are reviewed.

**Keywords:** Primary Sjögren's syndrome, central nervous system, multiple sclerosis-like disease

## Introduction

Sjögren's syndrome (SS) is a chronic autoimmune disorder mainly characterized by inflammatory damage of the exocrine glands, leading to reduced production of tears and saliva and consequently the symptoms of sicca syndrome. It is classified as primary Sjögren's syndrome (pSS) (also named only SS), in the absence of other associated autoimmune disorders, and secondary Sjögren's syndrome (sSS) (or associated SS) when linked usually with rheumatoid arthritis (RA), systemic lupus erythematosus (SLE) and systemic sclerosis (SSc). The spectrum of clinical presentation of pSS is highly variable, since multiple organ systems may also be affected. The majority of patients have symptoms of xerostomia and xerophthalmia (sicca syndrome) in association with minor systemic manifestations such as fatigue, myalgia, arthralgia and non-erosive polyarthritis. However, others develop serious organ involvements, including lymphocytic interstitial pneumonitis, cutaneous vasculitis, peripheral neuropathy, glomerulonephritis, optic neuritis, multiple sclerosis-like disease and even non-Hodgkin's B-cell lymphoma [1, 2]. In this chapter, we present a review on the central nervous system (CNS) damage in pSS concerning its frequency, pathogenesis, clinical manifestations, diagnosis, differential diagnosis and treatment. We begin with a brief review of the etiology, clinical features and classification criteria for pSS.

# Primary Sjögren's Syndrome

## Etiology

The etiology of pSS is unknown, but it is accepted that genetic susceptibility and environmental factors [i.e., Epstein-Barr virus (EBV)] contribute to the development of the disease [3]. Supporting this issue, EBV DNA was detected in epithelial cells from salivary [4, 5] and lacrimal glands [6] of pSS patients more often than in healthy individuals. In addition, the antibody to Epstein-Barr virus (EBV) early antigen diffuse (anti-EA-D), which is associated with viral replication, was detected in 36% of 100 pSS patients and in 4.5% of matched healthy control individuals ($p < 0.0001$) [7]. The concentrations of this reactivity also were significantly increased in the former group ($p<0.0001$). Interestingly, these findings were confirmed by assessing only the patients without current use of glucocorticoids and/or immunosuppressive agents, suggesting the possibility that a subclinical EBV reactivation may trigger or perpetuate the abnormal immune responses in pSS [7].

The autoimmune character of pSS is supported by the production of several circulating autoantibodies, primarily anti-Ro/SSA and anti-La/SSB [8, 9]. In this regard, there is evidence of molecular mimicry between EBV proteins with host antigens, particularly with Ro antigen, which could lead to an abnormal humoral immune response directed to self-antigens [10].

Indeed, pSS patients present an intense inflammatory infiltrate in the target tissues, particularly in the salivary and lacrimal glands, composed of activated T and B cells, dendritic cells, plasma cells and macrophages. The most remarkable histological feature of pSS is the periductal lymphocytic infiltrate in exocrine glands, which causes decreased glandular secretion. There is a predominance of activated CD4 helper T cells, which represent 60-70% of infiltrating lymphocytes [11]. These cells are critical in the pathogenesis of the disease, since they produce proinflammatory cytokines such as tumor necrosis factor-α (TNF-α) and interleukin-1 (IL-1) [12]. Cytokines are also produced by the activated epithelial cells in the salivary glands, and they play a crucial role in the development of pSS [13]. In this aspect, it was demonstrated recently enhanced regulation of the genes encoding interferon into cells in peripheral blood and salivary glands from pSS patients [14]. Interferon alpha (INFα) may stimulate the production of B-cell activating factor (BAFF), which improves maturation and differentiation of B lymphocytes. Supporting this notion, increased levels of BAFF were detected in salivary glands, saliva [15] and serum from pSS patients [16].

In its turn, B cells, which represent approximately 20% of the lymphocytic infiltrate in the salivary glands [11], produce multiple organ specific and non-organ specific autoantibodies, which may play a pathogenic role in the pSS [12].

In this regard, antibodies to muscarinic type 3 receptor (M3R) are detected in sera from pSS patients, and they may be an additional cause of decreased salivary flow, whose is stimulated by acetylcholine [17]. In addition, hypergammaglobulinemia, anti-Ro/SSA and anti-La/SSB antibodies and rheumatoid factor, striking features of pSS, indicate the presence of hyperactivity of B cells [18].

## Classification Criteria

Since the 1960s, approximately eleven recommendations for Sjögren's syndrome classification criteria were proposed by research groups. The classification criteria of the American-European Consensus Group were published in 2002, and they have been adopted by the majority of published studies on this disease, with more than 1,500 citations in the indexed literature (Table 1) [19].

In 2012, the American College of Rheumatology endorsed new criteria for SS classification proposed by the group Sjögren's International Collaborative Clinical Alliance (SICCA) [20]. These criteria are focused on three parameters: keratoconjunctivitis, sialoadenitis and serological features (Table 2).

The comparison between the two classification criteria shows that none of them is absolute. In fact, both have problems of sensitivity and specificity, because they depend on subjective considerations and clinical experience of the evaluator. This is due, at least in part, to the lack of knowledge about the mechanisms of disease, indicating that investment in research on the pathophysiology of Sjögren's syndrome is needed to address such questions [21].

**Table 1. American-European Consensus Group Criteria for Sjögren's Syndrome (2002)**

| |
|---|
| I. Ocular symptoms |
| II. Oral symptoms |
| III. Ocular signs- objective confirmation of ocular involvement defined as a positive result for at least one of the following tests: |
| Schimer's test (≤ 5 mm in 5 minutes). |
| Rose Bengal score or other dye score (≥ 4 according to van Bijsterveld's scoring system). |
| IV. Histopathology- in minor salivary glands, focal lymphocytic sialoadenitis, with a focus score ≥ 1, defined as the number of lymphocytic foci (which are adjacent to mucous acini and contain more than 50 lymphocytes) per 4 $mm^2$ of glandular tissue. |
| V. Salivary gland involvement- objective confirmation of salivary gland involvement defined by positive result for at least one of the: |
| Unstimulated salivary flow (≤ 1.5 ml in 15 minutes). |
| Parotid sialography showing the presence of diffuse sialectasias (punctate cavitary or destructive pattern), without evidence of obstruction in major ducts. |
| Salivary scintigraphy showing delayed uptake, reduced concentration and/or delayed excretion of tracer. |
| VI. Autoantibodies- presence in the serum of the following autoantibodies: |
| Antibodies to Ro/SSA and/or La/SSB antigens. |
| Primary Sjögren's syndrome is defined as: |
| (without any potentially associated systemic autoimmune disease) |
| The presence of any 4 of the 6 criteria, with either IV or VI. |
| The presence of any 3 of the 4 objective criteria (III, IV, V, VI). |
| Exclusion criteria: |
| Past head and neck radiation treatment. |
| Hepatitis C infection. |
| Acquired Immunodeficiency Syndrome (AIDS). |
| Pre-existing lymphoma. |
| Sarcoidosis. |
| Graft versus host disease. |
| Use of anticholinergic drugs. |

**Table 2. American College of Rheumatology 2012 Classification Criteria for Sjögren's Syndrome**

| |
|---|
| Keratoconjunctivitis sicca with ocular staining score ≥ 3 (without daily eye drops for glaucoma, corneal surgery or cosmetic eyelid surgery in the last 5 years). |
| Labial salivary gland biopsy with focal lymphocytic sialoadenitis (focus score≥ 1 focus/4 $mm^2$). |
| Positive anti-Ro/SSA and/or anti-La/SSB or positive rheumatoid factor and antinuclear antibodies (ANA) titre≥ 1:320. |
| Sjögren's syndrome is defined as: |
| In individuals with signs/symptoms suggestive of SS, at least 2 of the 3 objective above features. |
| Exclusion criteria: |
| History of head and neck radiation treatment. |
| Hepatitis C infection. |
| Acquired immunodeficiency syndrome. |
| Sarcoidosis. |
| Amyloidosis. |
| Graft versus host disease. |
| IgG4-related disease. |

## Epidemiology

The prevalence of pSS according to the American-European Consensus Group Criteria [19] is approximately 0.1-0.5% [22, 23]. The disease predominantly affects females (9:1), with a peak incidence between 40-60 years-old [8].

## Clinical Manifestations

The clinical characteristics of pSS may be basically divided into glandular and extraglandular manifestations. The most typical exocrinopathy in pSS is the sicca syndrome, xerophthalmia and xerostomia, which is due primarily to the destruction of glandular tissues by the inflammatory infiltrate. Reduction of salivary secretion leads to dryness of the oral mucosa, causing the symptoms of dry mouth, dysphagia for solid foods, multiple dental caries with tooth loss, oral candidiasis, disturbance of taste and atrophy of tongue papillae.

Enlargement of the parotid glands may also be observed on clinical examination [24]. Similarly, dry eye affects the corneal epithelium and may progress to keratoconjunctivitis sicca with corneal erosions and ulcers [25]. Patients may also present dry skin and dry vaginitis with dyspareunia [26].

On the other hand, extraglandular affections present a wide spectrum of clinical features (Table 3) [1, 8]. Systemic inflammation may cause constitutional symptoms such as fatigue, low grade fever, myalgia and arthralgia. The most common extraglandular manifestation is non-erosive polyarthritis of small and large joints. Cutaneous involvement is characterized by dry skin, Raynaud's phenomenon, annular erythema and vasculitis (mainly purpura in the lower limbs). The respiratory system may be affected causing dry cough due to xerotrachea, and dyspnea and hypoxemia resulting from damage of small airways, bronchiolitis and lymphocytic interstitial pneumonitis. Chronic atrophic gastritis with pernicious anemia, hepatomegaly and primary biliary cirrhosis may also occur. Kidney involvement is characterized by interstitial nephritis with renal tubular acidosis and, more rarely, membranous glomerulonephritis secondary to deposition of immune complexes. Peripheral neurological involvement may be due to vasa nervorum vasculitis, leading to sensorimotor polyneuropathy and mononeuritis multiplex. The involvement of central nervous systemic (CNS) is rare and may present as optic neuritis, myelitis and multiple sclerosis like-disease [1, 2, 8]. It is noteworthy that pSS patients have a risk for the development of lymphoma 18-44 times higher than the general population [27].

**Table 3. Major systemic manifestations in primary Sjögren's syndrome**

| Systemic manifestations | Frequencies (%) |
|---|---|
| Articular involvement | 37-75 |
| Raynaud's phenomenon | 16-48 |
| Cutaneous vasculitis | 11-12 |
| Pulmonary involvement | 23-37 |
| Kidney involvement | |
| Renal tubular acidosis | 6-9 |
| Glomerulonephritis | 1-2 |
| Peripheral neuropathy | 2-29 |
| Central nervous system involvement | 1-6 |
| Lymphoma | 2-4 |

# Nervous System Involvement

In primary Sjögren's syndrome, both central and peripheral nervous systems may be affected, and the prevalence of PNS and/or CNS involvement vary widely ranging from 0 to 70%, depending on the specific aspects of each study center (i.e., patients recruited from departments of internal medicine or neurology), the characteristics of the cohorts evaluated and also the different definitions and methods used for the diagnosis of neurological complications (i.e., whether or not including asymptomatic patients) [28, 29]. In addition, some case series have been evaluated before the establishment of the American-European Consensus Group Criteria (2002) for pSS classification, 2002 [19]. Most studies have reported a frequency of neurological complications in about 20% of cases [30-32].

Currently, there are no well-established criteria for definition of various neurological conditions described in association with the primary Sjögren's syndrome, which hampers the comparative analysis among the different published studies. Furthermore, it should be noted that most studies were carried out in referral centers, which may overestimate the prevalence of nervous system affection in pSS. The involvement of the peripheral nervous system (PNS) in pSS is a well-recognized condition in the literature, but the manifestations resulting from damage to the central nervous system (CNS) are considered rare, and they are still poorly understood regarding their pathogenesis, clinical presentation, diagnostic criteria and treatment [29].

Interestingly, neurological manifestations may precede the appearance of sicca symptoms in 40 to 93% of the cases [29], and the majority of patients are diagnosed with pSS after the neurological complication [31].

Then, we briefly review the pathogenesis and clinical features of the involvement of the peripheral nervous system, and we will focus in detail on the events concerning to the central nervous system damage in pSS.

## Peripheral Nervous System Involvement in Primary Sjögren's Syndrome

The involvement of the peripheral nervous system is considered the most common neurologic complication of primary Sjögren's syndrome by the majority of authors. PNS impairment in pSS is characterized mainly as sensory and sensorimotor axonal polyneuropathies (which represent over 50% of patients with PNS involvement), trigeminal neuropathy and small-fiber neuropathy [29, 33].

There are several hypotheses for the pathophysiological mechanism involved in the development of peripheral neurological symptoms, especially lymphocytic infiltration in the dorsal ganglion cells, causing ganglionitis, the vasa nervorum vasculitis, necrotizing vasculitis and participation of autoantibodies, such as antibodies to muscarinic receptors M3 and antineuronal antibodies, but the pathogenic role of these antibodies is still unknown [34-36].

The various manifestations resulting from peripheral nervous system involvement in pSS are as follows: axonal polyneuropathies (symmetric pure sensory peripheral neuropathy and symmetric sensorimotor peripheral neuropathy); sensory ganglioneuronopathy; motor neuropathy; small-fiber neuropathy; multiple mononeuritis; trigeminal and other cranial nerves neuropathies; autonomic neuropathies; and demyelinating polyradiculoneuropathy [37].

The axonal polyneuropathies are the most frequent clinical manifestations of PNS involvement in pSS. Early symptoms consist of distal symmetric sensory disorders in upper and lower limbs. The diagnosis is confirmed by the presence of large-fiber sensory dysfunction in the nerve conduction velocity studies and electromyography [33].

Recently, Brito-Zerón et al. retrospectively evaluated 563 consecutive pSS patients [37]. Peripheral neuropathies were classified into mononeuropathy, mononeuropathy multiplex, polyneuropathy and neuronopathy according to the electrodiagnostic studies. Nerve conduction studies were carried out in 158/563 (28%) pSS patients. The results were normal in 49 and abnormal in 109 patients, in whom peripheral neuropathy was diagnosed in 102. After excluding patients with neuropathy associated with other diseases and patients with entrapment mononeuropathies, 55/563 (10%) patients were classified as having SS-related peripheral neuropathy, including axonal sensorimotor polyneuropathy (n= 24), pure sensory neuronopathy (n= 15), mononeuropathy multiplex (n= 15) and demyelinating polyradiculoneuropathy (n= 1). In spite of therapy, clinical progression was observed in 12% of patients with axonal polyneuropathy, 13% of those with mononeuropathy multiplex and 47% of those with neuronopathy. Survival was significantly reduced in patients with peripheral neuropathy (especially in those with mononeuropathy multiplex and axonal polyneuropathy) in comparison with the control group [37].

Peripheral neuropathy does not usually respond well to treatment. Immunosuppressive therapy with glucocorticoids in high dosages, cyclophosphamide, azathioprine, and even plasmapheresis has shown only mild results [31, 33]. Rituximab, an anti-CD20 antibody, may be effective for the treatment of systemic manifestations in pSS patients [38], including some patients with refractory neuropathy [39]. In this regard, Mekinian et al. reported 17 pSS patients with PNS involvement treated with rituximab [40]. Neurological improvement occurred in 11 of 17 patients (65%) at three months, and the best responses were observed in patients with cryoglobulinemia or vasculitis (9 of 10 cases) [40].

## Central Nervous System Involvement in Primary Sjögren's Syndrome

### *Frequency and Clinical Presentations*

The frequency of central nervous system (CNS) involvement in pSS is still controversial, ranging from 0.3 to 48% [30, 41, 42]. However, it is considered an uncommon pSS systemic involvement by the most authors [8, 29]. Although uncommon, the CNS involvement in pSS may aggravate the patient's clinical condition and lead to motor and cognitive sequelae [42]. Furthermore, retrospective studies addressed to assess CNS injury in pSS suggest that the neurological manifestations are highly heterogeneous, often impairing their accurate diagnosis on clinical practice [33, 42].

In order to guide clinical practice, CNS manifestations in pSS may be classified according to Delalande et al. (2004) and Massara et al. (2010): focal/multifocal - motor and/or sensory deficits located in the territories of the brain, spinal cord and/or cerebellar syndrome; and diffuse - encephalopathy, psychosis, dementia and aseptic meningitis [33, 42]. Of note, some patients with multifocal lesions may be categorized with multiple sclerosis-like disease when the relapsing-remitting evolutive clinical course is comparable to MS. Optic neuritis may also be a focal neurological involvement in pSS. Neuromyelitis optica (NMO)-like syndrome may also affect these patients [33, 42].

The various manifestations resulting from central nervous system involvement in pSS are as follows: focal/multifocal (seizures, movement disorders, cerebellar syndrome, optic neuropathies, pseudotumor lesions, motor and sensory loss, multiple sclerosis-like disease and central nervous system vasculitic involvement); diffuse (cognitive impairment, encephalopathy, dementia, psychiatric abnormalities and (aseptic meningoencephalitis); and spinal cord dysfunction (acute and chronic progressive myelopathy, lower motor neuron disease, neurogenic bladder and acute transverse myelitis) [29].

In the series of Delalande et al. (2004), consisting of 56 pSS patients with CNS disorders referred to a neurologic department, CNS manifestations most commonly observed were focal or multifocal affections of the brain and/or spinal cord territories (≅ 100%), optic neuritis (23.2%), multiple sclerosis-like disease (17.9%), and primary multiple sclerosis (MS) (23.2%) [33]. Diffuse brain injuries, i.e., encephalopathy (2.4%) and cognitive disorders (11%) were rarely reported [33].

In contrast, Massara et al. (2010) found CNS disorders in 6% of 424 SS patients followed at a rheumatology unit, with predominance of diffuse manifestations (40%), including psychosis [42]. This discrepancy may be due to the peculiar characteristics of each reference center, as well as the inclusion of patients with different demographic and clinical features, besides the lack of a standardized classification for the CNS manifestations in pSS [33, 42].

In this respect, other authors consider headache and mood disorders as possible neurological affections of primary Sjögren's syndrome. Recently, Morreale et al. (2014) assessed 120 pSS patients [43]. All patients underwent to a neurological, neuropsychological, psychiatric, and neuroradiological evaluation. Central and peripheral nervous system involvement was observed in 81 patients (67.5%). The prevalence of CNS involvement was significantly higher than PNS disease (p= 0.001). Sixty-eight patients (84%) presented non-focal CNS symptoms and 64 (79%) focal CNS deficits with headache as the most common feature (46.9%), followed by cognitive (44.4%) and mood abnormalities (38.3%). These authors observed a high prevalence of migraine without aura, subcortical frontal executive functions and verbal memory impairment and apathy/alexythimia. Magnetic resonance spectroscopy (MRS) revealed a reduction of N-acetylaspartic acid (NAA) levels or NAA/creatine ratio decrease in subcortical frontal and basal ganglia white matter. At multivariate analysis, headache, cognitive disorders and psychiatric symptoms were significantly associated to serological markers (anti-Ro/SSA) and MRS characteristics. The association with immunological biomarkers and metabolic cerebral dysfunction suggests a possible endothelial dysfunction of the cerebral microvasculature or an inflammatory injury affecting nervous tissues [43].

Interestingly, ischemic stroke has rarely been described in women with Sjögren's syndrome without known traditional cardiovascular risk factors [44, 45]. In this regard, we evaluated 100 consecutive pSS patients and 89 age-gender-ethnicity-matched healthy controls for IgG/IgM anticardiolipin (aCL),

IgG/IgM anti-beta2-glycoprotein-I (aβ2GPI), and lupus anticoagulant (LA) [positivity according to antiphospholipid syndrome (APS) Sydney's criteria] [46]. Clinical analysis followed a standardized interview and physical examination assessing thrombotic and nonthrombotic APS manifestations and thrombosis risk factors. Antiphospholipid antibodies (aPLs) were detected in 16% patients and 5.6% controls ($p= 0.035$). LA was the most common aPL in pSS patients (9%), followed by aβ2GPI (5%) and aCL (4%). Thrombotic events occurred in five patients [stroke in two, myocardial infarction in one and deep-vein thrombosis (DVT) in four], but in none of controls ($p= 0.061$). Mean age at time of stroke was 35 years. Three patients with thrombotic events (including the two with stroke) had APS (Sydney's criteria) and were positive exclusively for LA. Comparison of patients with (n= 16) and without (n= 84) aPL revealed similar mean age, female predominance, and ethnicity ($p\geq 0.387$). Frequencies of livedo reticularis (25 vs. 4.8%, $p= 0.021$), stroke (12.5 vs. 0%, $p= 0.024$), and DVT (18.8 vs. 1.2%, $p= 0.013$) were significantly higher in APL positive patients. Conversely, frequencies of hypertension, dyslipidemia, diabetes, obesity, smoking, sedentarism, and hormonal contraception were similar in patients with or without aPL ($p\geq 0.253$). Our study identified LA as an important marker for APS in pSS, particularly for stroke in young patients, warranting routine evaluation of these antibodies and rigorous intervention in modifiable risk factors [46].

Pseudotumoral brain injury was also described in pSS [47]. It is important to highlight that compressive lesions are rare in pSS. Lymphoma and progressive multifocal leukoencephalopathy are differential diagnoses and both are possible complications of pSS [47].

### *Pathogenesis*

The pathogenic mechanisms responsible for the development of CNS injury in pSS are unknown. There are three hypotheses that may explain the pathophysiology of central dysfunctions: mononuclear infiltrate localized into the CNS [48]; vascular injury by antineuronal and anti-Ro/SSA antibodies [49]; and small vessel vasculitis causing ischemic tissue injury [50].

### *Risk Factors Associated to the Development of CNS Damage*

The possible risk factors associated with the development of this organ impairment are unknown. In this aspect, the available data suggest that longer disease duration, lung involvement and decreased serum levels of C4 were associated with CNS involvement in SS [42].

## Differential Diagnosis

Evaluating the case of a pSS patient with clinical manifestations suggestive of involvement of the central nervous system, we should be aware to the differential diagnosis especially with infectious disorders (encephalomyelitis and abscesses), hydroelectrolytic disturbances, neoplastic lesions (lymphoma, glioma and metastasis), progressive multifocal leukoencephalopathy, and other autoimmune diseases such as multiple sclerosis (MS) and optic neuromyelitis [29].

**Table 4. Differential diagnosis between multiple sclerosis and multiple sclerosis-like disease**

| | Multiple Sclerosis (MS) | Multiple Sclerosis-like disease |
|---|---|---|
| Anti-Ro/SSA<br>Anti-La/SSB | Negative in the majority of cases | Positive in the majority of cases |
| Anti-aquaporin-4 | Positive or negative | Negative in the majority of cases |
| Cerebrospinal fluid | Increased gamma globulin levels | Increased gamma globulin levels<br>Moderate lymphocyte pleocytosis |
| Oligoclonal bands | Present (3 or more) | Rarely |
| Magnetic nuclear resonance | Hyperintense areas in the subcortical and periventricular white matter on T2 and FLAIR. These lesions are more accentuated in MS, and they extend to the basal ganglia and the cerebral cortex.<br>Ovoid hypointense lesions in periventricular and justacortical areas on T1 ("black holes").<br>Spinal lesions ≤ 2 vertebral segments, only with partial cross sectional involvement of the spinal cord. | Hyperintense areas in the subcortical and periventricular white matter on T2 and FLAIR. |

Anti-aquaporin 4= neuromyelitis optica (NMO) IgG antibody.

In this regard, pSS has been diagnosed in series of MS patients in highly variable frequencies, of 4/440 (0.9%) [51] to 10/60 (16.7%) [52]. Additionally, pSS may mimic the clinical picture of MS and the differential diagnosis between these two diseases is sometimes challenging, especially in the initial presentations [53]. The presence of PNS involvement and older age are more suggestive of pSS than MS [41, 53]. In Table 4, we briefly present some laboratory and imaging features that may be helpful in the differential diagnosis between these two clinical conditions.

Another important aspect is the differential diagnosis with systemic lupus erythematosus (SLE), since secondary Sjögren's syndrome occur in up to 15% of these patients [54], and the non-exclusion of this confounding variable may reflect the known CNS involvement in SLE [55]. Thus, in addition to fulfillment of the international criteria for pSS [19] with exclusion of other connective tissue diseases, it is important to rule out the lupus-specific autoantibodies, anti-dsDNA, anti-Sm [56], and especially the anti-ribosomal P protein antibody (anti-Rib-P), which is associated with neuropsychiatric manifestations in SLE [57].

## Laboratory Tests and Imaging

The pSS patient with suspicion of CNS involvement should undergo complete medical history, clinical examination and neurological examination. In addition, the laboratory and imaging tests listed as follows may provide no specific evidence, but contribute to support diagnosis and differential diagnosis.

*Magnetic Resonance Imaging. (MRI):* MRI abnormalities are frequently observed in pSS patients, and generally consist in hyperintense areas in the subcortical and periventricular white matter on T2 and FLAIR [58] (Figure 1). Such areas are also present in patients with multiple sclerosis, but are more accentuated in the latter disease, and they extend to the basal ganglia and the cerebral cortex [29].

Furthermore, these lesions are not specific, and may be observed in patients with other autoimmune systemic diseases, such as systemic lupus erythematosus [59]. Their presence may indicate an underlying vascular inflammatory tissue injury [29], supporting previous hypotheses to explain the CNS damage in pSS, which includes the direct infiltration of the brain and/or spinal cord tissues by mononuclear cells and the ischemia secondary to small vessel vasculitis [29].

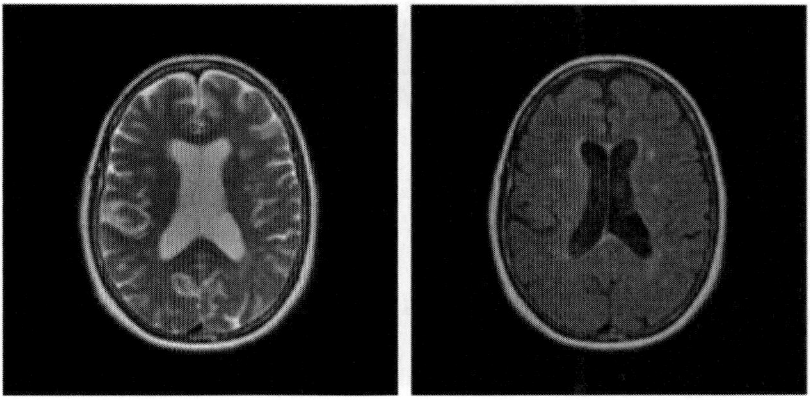

a b

Figure 1. Brain magnetic resonance imaging (MRI) on T2 (a) and FLAIR (b) from a pSS patient with multiple sclerosis-like disease. The MRI scan shows hyperintense lesions in the periventricular and subcortical white matter (WMH) on axial T2 (a) and axial image on FLAIR (b). Personal archive of the author.

*Cerebrospinal Fluid Analysis (CSF):* CSF is particularly useful for the differential diagnosis of infectious diseases. In aseptic meningoencephalitis, the cerebrospinal fluid characteristically shows high lymphocyte counts, increased levels of proteins and of gamma globulins [60]. CSF is also necessary for the differential diagnosis of multiple sclerosis. In this regard, oligoclonal bands (specifically more than three bands) are highly specific of multiple sclerosis. These bands have been reported in around 20% of pSS patients [61] and in over 90% in MS patients [62].

*Anti-aquaporin-4 (AQP4) antibody:* AQP4 is detected primarily in patients with neuromyelitis optica, but there is evidence of its presence in pSS [63]. Estiasari et al. (2012) observed positive AQP4 in 31.8% pSS patients [63]. The frequency of visual impairment was higher in anti-AQP4 antibody-positive patients than in antibody-negative patients (71.4% vs. 0.0%, p= 0.0008).

Brain MRI showed that discrete lesions were more commonly found in the cerebrum, brain stem, and optic nerve in anti-AQP4 antibody-positive patients than in antibody-negative patients (p= 0.002, p= 0.006, and p= 0.004, respectively), while spinal cord MRI showed that posterior column lesions in the cervical spinal cord were more frequent in anti-AQP4 antibody-positive patients than in antibody-negative patients (71.4% vs. 14.3%, p= 0.01). It is interesting that these clinical associations may represent an overlap of the diseases, pSS and neuromyelitis optica syndrome.

## Treatment

Due to the rarity and severity of central nervous system involvement in pSS, there is no established consensus for its therapeutic approach, with evidence resulting primarily from case reports and series of patients. Acute and chronic myelopathies are frequently severe and life-threatening. The response to glucocorticoid therapy ís generally poor. Treatment with cyclophosphamide plus high dosages of glucocorticoids has shown efficacy in some patients with CNS impairment, including myelopathies [29, 33, 64]. De Seze et al. demonstrated clinical response for acute and chronic myelopathies with the combination of glucorticoids and monthly intravenous cyclophosphamide [64]. Fourteen patients (6 with acute and 8 with chronic myelopathies) were evaluated. Nine patients improved clinically (including the 6 patients with acute myelopathy), three patients remained stable, and the other two patients presented progression of the neurological condition [64]. In fact, as a result of a systematic literature review, Ramos-Casals et al. punctuate that cyclophosphamide is the most frequently used immunosuppressive agent for the treatment of central nervous system involvement in pSS [65].

Recently, Mekinian et al. evaluated the efficacy of rituximab in treatment of CNS manifestations of pSS patients [66]. Prospective data from patients with pSS and CNS involvement included in the French Autoimmunity and Rituximab registry were analysed. All patients had diffuse white matter T2-weigted hypersignals. Neurological response was defined as improvement or disappearance of neurological signs. Eleven patients (mean age 55 years) were treated with rituximab for their neurological involvement. The mean duration of pSS was 9 years. Neurological features were progressive multiple sclerosis-like manifestations (n= 6), transverse myelitis (n= 1), anxiety and depression disorder (n= 1) and cognitive dysfunction (n= 3). The mean follow-up was of 13 months. No neurological change occurred in all 6 patients with multiple sclerosis-like symptoms, in 2/3 patients with cognitive dysfunction or in the patient with anxiety-depression. One patient with depression and cognitive dysfunction disclosed subjective improvement. One patient with transverse myelitis, refractory to cyclophosphamide had an improvement of his walk perimeter. These data suggest that rituximab does not seem to be effective in progressive multiple sclerosis-like disease of pSS patients [66], but larger studies are needed in this area.

## Conflict of Interests

The authors do not have any conflict of interest to declare.

## References

[1] Tzioufas, A.G.; Voulgarelis, M. Update on Sjögren's syndrome autoimmune epithelitis: from classification to increased neoplasias. *Best. Pract. Res. Clin. Rheumatol.* 2007; 21: 989-1010.

[2] Amarasena, R.; Bowman, S. Sjögren's syndrome. *Clin. Med.* 2007; 7: 53-56.

[3] Toussirot, E.; Roudier, J. Epstein-Barr virus in autoimmune diseases. *Best. Pract. Res. Clin. Rheumatol.* 2008; 22: 883-896.

[4] Mariette, X.; Gozlan, J.; Clerc, D.; Bisson, M.; Morinet, F. Detection of Epstein-Barr virus DNA by in situ hybridization and polymerase chain reaction in salivary gland biopsy specimens from patients with Sjögren's syndrome. *Am. J. Med.* 1991; 90: 286-294.

[5] Perrot, S.; Calvez, V.; Escande, J.P.; Dupin, N.; Marcelin, A.G. Prevalences of herpesviruses DNA sequences in salivary gland biopsies from primary and secondary Sjögren's syndrome using degenerated consensus PCR primers. *J. Clin. Virol.* 2003; 28: 165-168.

[6] Pflugfelder, S.C.; Crouse, C.; Pereira, I.; Atherton, S. Amplification of Epstein-Barr virus genomic sequences in blood cells, lacrimal glands, and tears from primary Sjögren's syndrome patients. *Ophthalmology* 1990; 97: 976-984.

[7] Pasoto S.G.; Natalino R.R.; Chakkour, H.P.; et al. EBV reactivation serological profile in primary Sjögren's syndrome: an underlying trigger of active articular involvement? *Rheumatol. Int.* 2013; 33: 1149-1157.

[8] García-Carrasco, M.; Ramos-Casals, M.; Rosas, J.; et al. Primary Sjögren syndrome: clinical and immunologic disease patterns in a cohort of 400 patients. *Medicine* 2002; 81: 270-280.

[9] Nardi, N.; Brito-Zerón, P.; Ramos-Casals, M.; et al. Circulating auto-antibodies against nuclear and non-nuclear antigens in primary Sjögren's syndrome. Prevalence and clinical significance in 335 patients. *Clin. Rheumatol.* 2006; 25: 341-346.

[10] Poole, B.D.; Scofield, R.H.; Harley, J.B.; James, J.A. Epstein-Barr virus and molecular mimicry in systemic lupus erythematosus. *Autoimmunity* 2006; 39: 63-70.

[11] Fox, R.I.; Adamson, T.C. 3rd; Fong, S.; Young, C.; Howell, F.V. Characterization of the phenotype and function of lymphocytes infiltrating the salivary gland in patients with primary Sjogren syndrome. *Diagn. Immunol.* 1983; 1: 233-239.

[12] Delaleu, N.; Jonsson, M.V.; Appel, S.; Jonsson, R. New concepts in the pathogenesis of Sjögren's syndrome. *Rheum. Dis. Clin. N. Am.* 2008; 34: 833-845.

[13] Chiorini, J.A.; Cihakova, D.; Ouellette, C.E.; Caturegli, P. Sjögren syndrome: advances in the pathogenesis from animal models. *J. Autoimmun.* 2009; 33: 190-196.

[14] Nikolov, N.P.; Illei, G.G. Pathogenesis of Sjögren's syndrome. *Curr. Opin. Rheumatol.* 2009; 21: 465-470.

[15] Lavie, F.; Miceli-Richard, C.; Quillard, J.; Roux, S.; Leclerc, P.; Mariette, X. Expression of BAFF (BLyS) in T cells infiltrating labial salivary glands from patients with Sjögren's syndrome. *J. Pathol.* 2004; 202: 496-502.

[16] Lavie, F.; Miceli-Richard, C.; Ittah, M.; Sellam, J.; Gottenberg, J.E.; Mariette, X. B-cell activating factor of the tumor necrosis factor family expression in blood monocytes and T cells from patients with primary Sjögren's syndrome. *Scand. J. Immunol.*2008; 67: 185-192.

[17] Kovács, L.; Fehér, E.; Bodnár, I.; et al. Demonstration of autoantibody binding to muscarinic acetylcholine receptors in the salivary gland in primary Sjögren's syndrome. *Clin. Immunol.* 2008; 128: 269-276.

[18] Routsias, J.G.; Tzioufas, A.G. Sjögren's syndrome- study of autoantigens and autoantibodies. *Clinic. Rev. Allerg. Immunol.* 2007; 32: 238-251.

[19] Vitali, C.; Bombardieri, S.; Jonsson, R.; et al. Classification criteria for Sjögren's syndrome: a revised version of the European criteria proposed by the American-European Consensus Group. *Ann. Rheum. Dis.* 2002; 61: 554-558.

[20] Shiboski, S.C.; Shiboski, C.H.; Criswell, L.; et al. American College of Rheumatology classification criteria for Sjögren's syndrome: a data-driven, expert consensus approach in the Sjögren's International Collaborative Clinical Alliance cohort. *Arthritis Care Res. (Hoboken)* 2012; 64: 475-487.

[21] Rasmussen, A.; Ice, J.A.; Li, H.; et al. Comparison of the American-European Consensus Group Sjogren's syndrome classification criteria to newly proposed American College of Rheumatology criteria in a large, carefully characterised sicca cohort. *Ann. Rheum. Dis.* 2014; 73: 31-38.

[22] Bowman, S.J.; Ibrahim, G.H.; Holmes, G.; Hamburguer, J.; Ainsworth, J. Estimating the prevalence among Caucasian women of primary Sjögren's syndrome in two general practices in Birmingham, UK. *Scand. J. Rheumatol.* 2004; 33: 39-43.

[23] Sánchez-Guerrero, J.; Pérez-Dosal, M.R.; Cárdenas-Velázquez, F.; et al. Prevalence of Sjögren's syndrome in ambulatory patients according to the American-European Consensus Group criteria. *Rheumatology* 2005; 44: 235-240.

[24] Bayetto, K.; Logan, R.M. Sjogren's syndrome: a review of aetiology, pathogenesis, diagnosis and management. *Aust. Dent. J.* 2010; 55 (1 Suppl): 39-47.

[25] Mohsenin, A.; Huang, J.J. Ocular manifestations of systemic inflammatory diseases. *Conn. Med.* 2012; 76: 533-544.

[26] Venables, P.J. Sjögren's syndrome. *Best. Pract. Res. Clin. Rheumatol.* 2004; 18: 313-329.

[27] Voulgarelis, M.; Moutsopoulos, H.M. Mucosa-associated lymphoid tissue lymphoma in Sjögren's syndrome: risks, management and prognosis. *Rheum. Dis. Clin. N. Am.* 2008; 34: 921-933.

[28] Chai, J.; Logigian, E.L. Neurological manifestations of primary Sjögren's syndrome. *Curr. Opin. Neurol.* 2010; 23: 509-513.

[29] Tobón, G.J.; Pers, J.O.; Devauchelle-Pensec, V.; Youinou, P. Neurological disorders in primary Sjögren's syndrome. *Autoimmune Dis.* 2012; 2012: 645967.

[30] Govoni, M.; Padovan, M.; Rizzo, N.; Trotta, F. CNS involvement in primary Sjögren's syndrome: prevalence, clinical aspects, diagnostic assessment and therapeutic approach. *CNS Drugs* 2001; 15: 597-607.

[31] Mori, K.; Iijima, M.; Koike, H., et al. The wide spectrum of clinical manifestations in Sjögren's syndrome-associated neuropathy. *Brain* 2005; 128: 2518-2534.

[32] Goransson, L.G.; Herigstad, A.; Tjensvoll, A.B.; Harboe, E.; Mellgren, S.I.; Omdal, R. Peripheral neuropathy in primary Sjögren's syndrome: a population-based study. *Arch. Neurol.* 2006; 63: 1612-1615.

[33] Delalande, S.; De Seze, J.; Fauchais, A.L.; et al. Neurologic manifestations in primary Sjögren syndrome: a study of 82 patients. *Medicine* 2004; 83: 280-291.

[34] Malinow, K.; Yannakakis, G.D.; Glusman, S.M., et al. Subacute sensory neuronopahty secondary to dorsal root ganglionitis in primary Sjögren's syndrome. *Ann. Neurol.* 1986; 20: 535-537.

[35] Mellgren, S.I.; Conn, D.L.; Stevens, J.C.; Dyck, P.J. Peripheral neuropathy in primary Sjögren's syndrome. *Neurology* 1989; 39: 390-394.

[36] Murata, Y.; Maeda, K.; Hawai, H.; et al. Antiganglion neuron antibodies correlate with neuropathy in Sjögren's syndrome. *Neuro. Report.* 2005; 16: 677-681.

[37] Brito-Zerón, P.; Akasbi, M.; Bosch, X., et al. Classification and characterisation of peripheral neuropathies in 102 patients with primary Sjögren's syndrome. *Clin. Exp. Rheumatol.* 2013; 31: 103-110.

[38] Seror, R.; Sordet, C.; Guillevin, L.; et al. Tolerance and efficacy of rituximab and changes in serum B cell biomarkers in patients with systemic complications of primary Sjögren's syndrome. *Ann. Rheum. Dis.* 2007; 66: 351-357.

[39] Gorson, K.C.; Natarajan, N.; Ropper, A.H.; Weinstein, R. Rituximab treatment in patients with IVIg-dependent immune polyneuropathy: a prospective pilot trial. *Muscle and Nerve* 2007; 35: 66-69.

[40] Mekinian, A.; Ravaud, P.; Hatron, P.Y., et al. Efficacy of rituximab in primary Sjögren's syndrome with peripheral nervous system involvement: results from the AIR registry. *Ann. Rheum. Dis.* 2011; 71: 84-87.

[41] Soliotis, F.C.; Mavragani, C.P.; Moutsopoulos, H.M. Central nervous system involvement in Sjögren's syndrome. *Ann. Rheum. Dis.* 2004; 63: 616-620.

[42] Massara, A.; Bonazza, S.; Castellino, G., et al. Central nervous system involvement in Sjögren's syndrome: unusual, but not unremarkable – clinical, serological characteristics and outcomes in a large cohort of Italian patients. *Rheumatology* 2010; 49: 1510-1549.

[43] Morreale, M.; Marchione, P.; Giacomini, P.; et al. Neurological involvement in primary Sjögren syndrome: a focus on central nervous system. *PloS One* 2014; 9: e84605.

[44] Bragoni, M.; Di Piero, V.; Priori, R.; Valesini, G., Lenzi, GL. Sjögren's syndrome presenting as ischemic stroke. *Stroke* 1994; 25: 2276-2279.

[45] Koh, M.S.; Goh, K.Y.; Chen, C.; Howe, H.S. Cerebral infarct mimicking glioma in Sjogren's syndrome. *Hong Kong Med. J.* 2002; 8: 292-294.

[46] Pasoto, S.G.; Chakkour, H.P.; Natalino, R.R., et al. Lupus anticoagulant: a marker for stroke and venous thrombosis in primary Sjögren's syndrome. *Clin. Rheumatol.* 2012; 31: 1331-1338.

[47] Sassi, S.B.; Nabli, F.; Boubaker, A., et al. Pseudotumoral brain lesion as the presenting feature of primary Sjögren's syndrome. *J. Neurol. Sci.* 2004; pii: S0022-510X(14)00051-3.

[48] Bakchin, S.; Duyckaerts, C.; Hassine, K., et al. Central and peripheral neurologic lesions in primary Gougerot-Sjögren syndrome. Clinicopathological study of a case. *Rev. Neurol.* 1991; 147: 368-375.

[49] Alexander, E.L.; Ranzenbach, M.R.; Kumar, A.J.; et al. Anti-Ro(SS-A) autoantibodies in central nervous system disease associated with Sjögren's syndrome: clinical, neuroimaging and angiographic correlates. *Neurology* 1994; 44: 899-908.

[50] Alexander, E.L.; Provost, T.T.; Sanders, M.E.; Frank, M.; Joiner, K.A. Serum complement activation in central nervous system disease in Sjögren's syndrome. *Am. J. Med.* 1988; 85: 513-518.

[51] Annunziata, P.; De Santi, L.; Di Rezze, S.; et al. Clinical features of Sjogren's syndrome in patients with multiple sclerosis. *Acta Neurol. Scand.* 2011; 124: 109-114.

[52] de Seze, J.; Devos, D.; Castelnovo, G.; et al. The prevalence of Sjögren syndrome in patients with primary progressive multiple sclerosis. *Neurology* 2001; 57: 1359-1363.

[53] Eckstein, C.; Saidha, S; Levy, M. A differential diagnosis of central nervous system demyelination: beyond multiple sclerosis. *J. Neurol.* 2012; 259: 801-816.

[54] Theander, E.; Jacobsson, L.T. Relationship of Sjögren's syndrome to other connective tissue and autoimmune disorders. *Rheum. Dis. Clin. North Am.* 2008; 34: 935-947.

[55] Bertsias, G.K.; Ioannidis, J.P.; Aringer, M.; et al. EULAR recommendations for the management of systemic lupus erythematosus with neuropsychiatric manifestations: report of a task force of the EULAR standing committee for clinical affairs. *Ann. Rheum. Dis.* 2010; 69: 2074-2082.

[56] Tan, E.M. Autoantibodies, autoimmune disease, and the birth of immune diagnostics. *J. Clin. Invest.* 2012; 122: 3835-3836.

[57] Reichlin, M. Autoantibodies to the ribosomal P proteins in systemic lupus erythematosus. *Clin. Exp. Med.* 2006; 6: 49-52.

[58] Morgen, K.; McFarland, H.F.; Pillemer, S.R. Central nervous system disease in primary Sjögren's syndrome: the role of magnetic resonance imaging. *Sem. Arthritis Rheum.* 2004; 34: 623-630.

[59] Rovaris, M.; Inglese, M.; Viti, B.; et al. The contribution of fast-FLAIR MRI for lesion detection in the brain of patients with systemic autoimmune diseases. *J. Neurol.* 2000; 247: 29-33.

[60] Lafitte, C. Neuroradiological manifestations of primary Sjögren's syndrome. *Rev. Neurol.* 2002; 158: 959-965.

[61] Vrethem, M.; Ernerudh, J.; Lindstrom, F.; Skogh, T. Immunoglobulins within the central nervous system in primary Sjögren's syndrome. *J. Neurol. Sci.* 1990; 100: 186-192.

[62] Bourahoui, A.; De Seze, J.; Guttierez, R., et al. CSF isoelectrofocusing in a large cohort of MS and other neurological diseases. *Eur. J. Neurol.* 2004; 11: 525-529.

[63] Estiasari, R.; Matsushita, T.; Masaki, K., et al.. Comparison of clinical, immunological and neuroimaging features between anti-aquaporin-4 antibody-positive and antibody-negative Sjogren's syndrome patients with central nervous system manifestations. *Mult. Scler.* 2012; 18: 807-816.

[64] De Seze, J.; Delalande, S.; Fauchais, A.L., et al. Myelopathies secondary to Sjögren's syndrome: treatment with monthly intravenous cyclophosphamide associated with corticosteroids. *J. Rheumatol.* 2006; 33: 709-711.

[65] Ramos-Casals, M.; Brito-Zerón, P.; Sisó-Almirall, A.; et al. Topical and systemic medications for the treatment of primary Sjögren's syndrome. *Nat. Rev. Rheumatol.* 2012; 8: 399-411.

[66] Mekinian, A.; Ravaud, P.; Larroche, C.; et al. Rituximab in central nervous system manifestations of patients with primary Sjögren's syndrome: results from the AIR registry. *Clin. Exp. Rheumatol.* 2012; 30: 208-212.

In: Sjögren's Syndrome
Editor: Eduardo M. Hernandez
ISBN: 978-1-63117-859-7


*Chapter VI*

# New Aspects of Mechanism of Salivary Gland Dysfunction in Sjögren's Syndrome

***Takashi Fujimoto*[1], *Kiyomi Yoshimoto*[2], *Takanori Fujimura*[1,3], *Maiko Takeda*[3], *Asako Itaya-Hironaka*[3] *and Shin Takasawa*[3*]**

[1]The Center for Rheumatic Diseases
[2] Department of General Medicine
[3] Department of Biochemistry,
Nara Medical University, Kashihara, Japan

## Abstract

Sjögren's syndrome, an autoimmune disease characterized by exocrine gland dysfunction leading to dry mouth and dry eye diseases, is typified by lymphoplasmacytic infiltrations and a progressive destruction of the salivary and lacrimal glands. Despite an ever-increasing focus on identifying the underlying etiology of Sjögren's syndrome, defining factors that initiate this autoimmune disease and mechanisms that develop the following exocrine gland dysfunction remain a mystery.

* Correspondence: Prof. Shin Takasawa, Department of Biochemistry, Nara Medical University, 840 Shijo-cho, Kashihara 634-8521, Nara, Japan; Tel: 81-744-22-3051 Ext. 2227; FAX: 81-744-24-9525; E-mail: shintksw@naramed-u.ac.jp.

The original explanatory concept for the pathogenesis of Sjögren's syndrome proposed a specific, self-perpetuating, immune mediated loss of acinar and ductal cells as the principal cause of salivary gland dysfunction. Accordingly, apoptosis, fibrosis and atrophy of the salivary glands would represent consequences of salivary gland hypofunction.

In this chapter we highlight the possible involvement of **re**generating **g**ene (*Reg*) in regeneration and destruction of salivary gland acinar and ductal cells in Sjögren's syndrome. *Reg* gene was originally isolated as a gene specifically overexpressed in regenerating pancreatic islets and constitute a growth factor family (Reg family). *Reg* gene product (Reg protein) is important in the pathophysiology of various human inflammatory diseases such as diabetes, inflammatory bowel disease(s), and Sjögren's syndrome. We describe how the salivary gland dysfunction is initiated and maintained, and how it can be regenerated or progressed mediated by *Reg* gene and Reg protein. We also touch on recent aspects of potential molecular mechanisms underlying immune-mediated salivary gland dysfunction prior to glandular destruction and atrophy, resulting in the symptoms of dryness in Sjögren's syndrome.

# Introduction

Sjögren's syndrome is a chronic inflammatory disease that affects the exocrine glands, particularly salivary and lacrimal glands, leading to xerostomia and xerophthalmia, and characterized by the presence of a variety autoantibodies directed against organ and non-organ-specific autoantigens. Focal, mononuclear cell infiltrates surround the ducts and replace the secretory units. Primary Sjögren's syndrome is a common systemic auto immune disorder, affecting approximately 0.1–0.4% of the general population with a female to male ratio of 9:1, a prevalence that is comparable to that of rheumatoid arthritis [1–6]. It is known that the production of autoantibodies is an antigen-driven immune response, as certain autoantibodies are disease-specific, contain multiple epitopes and the autoimmune response is perpetuated and augmented via intra- and intermolecular spreading against the same or other autoantigens. It is unknown whether or not any of the autoantibodies has a direct pathogenic potential or they merely participate in a secondary response to salivary glands that are already damaged by another process. Although the pathogenetic mechanisms of this autoimmune exocrinopathy are not yet fully known, Sjögren's syndrome arises either as the primary disease or occurring secondary to other autoimmune rheumatic diseases as a result of infiltration of the functional glandular epithelium by autoreactive lymphocytes [7]. The original explanatory concept for the pathogenesis of Sjögren's syndrome proposed a specific, self-perpetuating, immune mediated loss of acinar and ductal cells as the principal cause of salivary gland dysfunction. Accordingly, apoptosis, fibrosis and atrophy of the salivary glands would represent consequences of salivary gland hypofunction.

In this chapter, we aim to describe important pathogenetic mechanisms involved in the initiation and perpetuation of Sjögren's syndrome. In particular, we highlight the possible involvement of **re**generating **g**ene (*Reg*) in regeneration and destruction of salivary gland acinar and ductal cells in Sjögren's syndrome.

## Pathogenesis of Sjögren's Syndrome

As previously mentioned, the pathogenetic mechanisms responsible for Sjögren's syndrome are not yet fully known, but in the presence of a susceptible genetic background, both environmental and hormonal factors are thought to be capable of triggering this autoimmune exocrinopathy. Salivary, lacrimal, and other exocrine glands become infiltrated with CD4+ T cells, but substantial numbers of B lymphocytes and plasma cells are also present in inflamed tissues. Moreover, glandular alteration in cell migration can also lead to the formation of germinal center like structures that contain follicular dendritic cells and proliferating B lymphocytes [8, 9]. During the past 15 years, the importance of the epithelial cell in the pathogenesis and evolution of Sjögren's syndrome has been highlighted and has prompted the use of the term'autoimmune epithelitis'as an alternative name for the disease [10].

Immunologically-activated or apoptotic glandular epithelial cells that expose autoantigens in genetically predisposed individuals might drive autoimmune-mediated tissue injury. Critical to the initiation and perpetuation of Sjögren's syndrome pathogenesis are the upregulation of adhesion molecules and the production of chemokines and cytokines, which together promote the migration of lymphocytes and dendritic cells into the glands, maintaining their cycle of homing.

Extension of the pathological process that affects the exocrine glands into periepithelial and extraepithelial tissue can cause a considerable percentage of patients to exhibit systemic findings that involve the lungs, liver or kidneys. These manifestations develop as a result of lymphocytic invasion or an immune-complex mediated process, or both, and present as skin vasculitis coupled with peripheral neuropathy or glomerulonephritis.

# Previous Research

Apoptosis, nonapoptosis, and abnormal distribution/expression of aquaporin before the inflammation, will be introduced. Afterwards cytokines and acquired immunity will be also included.

## 1. Apoptosis/ Nonapoptosis

Classically, the pathogenesis of Sjögren's syndrome proposed in explaining glandular hypofunction is a two-step mechanism. At first, a primary immune attack by infiltrating lymphocytes and at second cytotoxic cell death (necrosis) and apoptosis, which may be one of factors relating with dysfunction of salivary and lacrimal glands, in genetically predisposed individuals may occur [11]. Some reports of apoptosis induced probably by genetic abnormality including the role of apoptosis as initiator will be introduced. Also, opposite opinions against apoptosis in general pathogenetic roles are included. It has been demonstrated using non-obese diabetic (NOD) mice and NOD scid (immunodeficient) mice that the pathogenesis of Sjögren's syndrome occurs in two phases: an asymptomatic phase epithelial cells of exocrine tissues undergo dedifferentiation accompanied by elevated apoptosis and a second phase in which autoimmunity is mounted against target organ autoantigens, resulting in the activation of T and B lymphocytes, and the generation of autoantibodies [12]. Humphreys-Beher et al. [13] reported that genetic alterations in glandular homeostasis involving the death program may contribute to disease progression or even in the initial trigger of autoimmunity, since there are high levels of apoptosis and aberrant protein expression in the submandibular gland in the absence of an immune response in NOD mice. Kong et al. [14] demonstrated that apoptosis of the secretory epithelial cells occurs in both NOD and NOD-scid mice in salivary and lacrimal glands in which Fas protein and mRNA were expressed only in the exocrine glands before inflammation in NOD and NOD-scid mice, but not in normal BALB/c mice. A potential apoptotic process dependent on Fas/Fas ligand (FasL) interactions occurring in NOD-scid glandular secretory epithelial cells strongly suggests the apoptosis may precede lymphocytic infiltration [14]. Qi et al. [15] reported that apoptosis may be initiator of inflammation in target organs in which lacrimal dysfunction was found in the early age without inflammation in NOD mice, and apoptotic cells exist in acinar epithelium at 5 weeks of age, but not 2 weeks of age without inflammatory foci in submandibular glands. If that is the case, apoptosis may be induced genetically as well as immunologically. The relationship between apoptosis and dysfunction of glands in NOD-scid mice is unclear. Apoptosis before inflammation in human Sjögren's syndrome is not known.

Apoptosis of the epithelial cells in the salivary glands has been shown to be a rare event [16]. Many patients with Sjögren's syndrome who have little or no glandular function (as evidenced by markedly diminished or absent saliva output) retain large amounts of normal-appearing acinar tissue in their salivary glands [17]. This residual tissue is functional in vitro [18, 19], although they show a reduced sensitivity to muscarinic stimulation [19]. Van Blokland et al. [20] reported that before and after the onset of sialoadenitis in NOD and NOD-scid mice, numbers of apoptotic cells were not increased as compared with control mice at any age. Nonapoptosis mechanisms before inflammation do not deny the role of apoptosis during the process of inflammation, since there are a number of references that apoptosis may play an important role in the pathogenesis of Sjögren's syndrome [21], but there is a possibility of non-apoptotic mechanisms during the process of the disease. Using a non-apoptotic model for glandular hypofunction, Dawson et al. [21] have suggested that interaction between the immune system and the secretory process could lead to glandular hypofunction such as inhibition of neurotransmitter release by cytokines, enhanced breakdown of acethylcoline (ACh) by increased levels of cholinesterase, blockade of ACh receptor M3 (M3R) by antimuscarinic autoantibodies, and altered expression or distribution of aquaporin5.

## 2. Aquaporin

Fundamental importance of aquaporins by their conservation from bacteria through plants to mammals has been suggested, and ten mammalian aquaporins (AQPs) identified are expressed in several organs (e.g., the kidney, lung, eye, and brain) and multiple water-channel proteins that regulate the movement of water through the plasma membrane of secretory and absorptive cells in response to osmotic gradients [22]. In this section, at first normal distribution/expression of AQPs in healthy human and animals will be mentioned. Also abnormal distribution/ expression of AQPs from human Sjögren's syndrome, who may have inflammation, and then data from mice will be introduced. Abnormal distribution and expression of aquaporin 5 (AQP5) in acini of salivary glands are likely to contribute to the deficiency of fluid secretion during the noninflammatory phase but also during the immunologic phase. Recently, it has been reported in more details that AQP5 appeared mainly at the apical membrane of mucous glands, basolateral membrane, and basal membrane of serous acini including intense staining in the intercalated ducts, striated ducts, and secretory ducts of the labial gland in healthy volunteers, whereas AQP5 was distributed at the basal membrane and obviously reduced at the apical membrane in patients with Sjögren's syndrome (Figure 1) [23, 24].

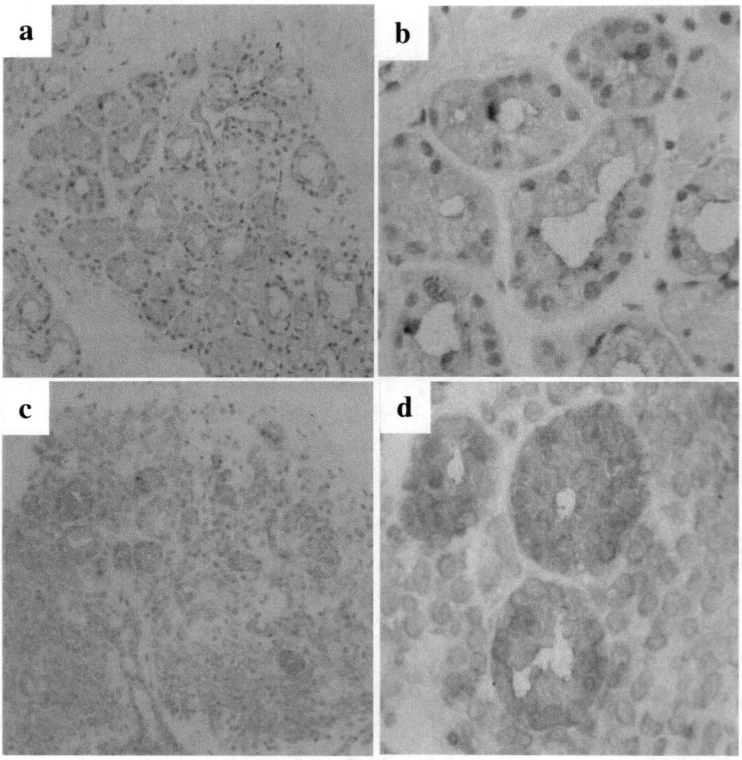


Figure 1. Immunohistochemical localization of human AQP5 in MSG (adopted from [24]). Human AQP5 was localized on MSG sections from a control subject (a, b), a Sjögren's syndrome patient with severe lymphoid infiltration (c, d). Indirect immunofluorescence staining using affinity-purified human AQP5 antibodies was performed. In MSG biopsy specimens from control subjects, almost of all AQP5 was detected at the apical membrane of the acinar cell (a, b). In contrast, in MSG biopsy specimens from Sjögren's syndrome patients, human AQP5 was not predominantly localized to the apical membrane of the acinar cell but diffusely expressed at the cytoplasm (apical, basolateral and intracellular) of the acinar cell (c, d).

Among AQPs, AQP5 seems to be the only AQP playing a major role in the salivary secretion process and its expression was higher at the basal membrane, and lower at the apical membrane of acinar cells of salivary gland in primary Sjögren's syndrome (pSS) [25]. Patients with pSS or secondary Sjögren's syndrome (sSS) showing high percentage of reactivity of acinus area with AQP5 revealed AQP5 primarily at the basal membranes of the acinus, whereas in patients with low percentage of acinus area AQP5 was detected at the apical membrane of acinar cells of salivary gland in patients with pSS [26]. Tsubota et al. [27] reported cytoplasmic AQP5 was seen in patients with SS. Abnormal distribution/expression of AQP5 in acinar epithelium of minor salivary glands lacking inflammatory cell infiltration was observed, suggesting that their abnormal expression may not be due to only direct inflammatory cell reaction, even in the inflammatory phase [28]. By the comparative study between AQP5+/+ mouse and AQP5 knockout (AQP5-/-) mouse AQP5 was localized mainly in the ductal cells rather than in the acinar cells of the lacrimal gland without decreased tear secretion, whereas in the parotid gland AQP5 was observed abundantly in acinar cells, but not in ductal cells, with reduced saliva secretion [29]. In addition, Krane et al. [30] reported that water permeability decreased by 65% in parotid and 77% in sublingual acinar cells from AQP5-/- mice in response to hypertonicity-induced cell shrinkage and hypotonicity-induced cell swelling. These data show that AQP5 is the major pathway for regulating the water permeability in parotid and sublingual acinar cells (a critical property of the plasma membrane which determines the flow rate and ionic composition of secreted saliva). Soyfoo et al. [31] reported that the 8-week-old female NOD mice without inflammation and normal age-matched BALB/c (normal) mice showed a similar distribution of AQP5 primarily at the apical membrane of the salivary gland acini, whereas in acini from the submandibular glands (but not from the parotid glands) from 24-week-old NOD mice with inflammation, AQP5 staining was reduced at the apical membrane but was increased at the basal membrane compared to normal mice, in which a significant decrease in pilocarpine-stimulated salivary flow was observed. On the other hand, Nishimura et al. [32] reported that AQP5 was expressed in the apical and lateral cell membranes of acinar cells in the parotid and submandibular glands of normal mice, but not in the sublingual glands, whereas AQP5 was expressed not only in the cell membranes of acinar cells in the apical domains but also in the cytoplasm in the female MRL/lpr mouse, a model for not only rheumatoid arthritis (RA)-like disease but also sSS in human. There are some differences in distribution/expression of AQPs. Thus, it has been pointed out that the hypothesis that AQP5 has a major role in the pathogenesis of pSS needs to be reassessed and unconfirmed issue has to be determined [33]. However, accumulating evidence suggests that abnormal AQP5 expression/distribution in acinar epithelium of salivary (especially submandibular) glands, at least, may contribute to hyposalivation at some extent before inflammation.

## 3. Type I Interferon / Cytokine

Type I interferon (IFN) will be introduced in this section from the point of innate immunity before the development of immune reaction. Regarding the role of type I IFN, studies in human Sjögren's syndrome are relatively well done. Current trends in autoimmune diseases are focusing on innate immunity, which acts as a trigger on multiple autoimmune diseases [34]. Type I IFN will be produced as a consequence of the development of innate immunity. High values of type I IFN are rapidly produced in viral infection [35], but also in autoimmune diseases such as systemic lupus erythematosus (SLE) [36]. Serum levels of type I IFN were found to be high in pSS patients compared with normal individuals reported by some groups [37, 38], but not by others [39]. Other than role of type I IFN, the central role of B cell-activating factor (BAFF), which promotes B cell survival and exists in a membrane bound and a secreted form, has been reported in pSS [40]. BAFF production and its mRNA expression by cultured human minor salivary gland (MSG) epithelial cells obtained from pSS patients can be upregulated after stimulation by chemical Toll like receptors (TLRs) agonist (Poly I:C) or viruses such as retrovirus type I through pathways dependent on TLRs and independent of type I IFN [40]. Moreover, in systemic autoimmune diseases such as SLE environmental factors (e.g., viral infections), and apoptotic bodies and immune complexes stimulate plasmacytoid dendritic cells (pDCs) through coengagement of the TLRs and Fc$\gamma$ receptor, resulting in the production of type I IFN from pDCs. Thereafter, type I IFN induces the generation of immunogenic mature DCs, resulting in suppression of regulatory T (Treg) cell function, which maintain self-tolerance [41, 42]. Alternatively, TLR3 activation associated with type I IFN upregulation led to rapid onset and reversible hyposalivation without glandular inflammation [43], suggesting that salivary gland dysfunction may precede autoimmunity development or represent a separate process in the pathogenesis of Sjögren's syndrome. It is reported using global gene expression profiling that locally produced IFN$\alpha$ is detected at higher levels in acini and endothelial cells compared with controls, but IFN$\alpha$ is mainly secreted by pDCs, which are found in the salivary glands of pSS patients but not in healthy controls [44]. Thus, IFN-$\alpha$ in circulation in pSS is argued, since serum IFN$\alpha$ was detected in very few people with pSS [45-47], suggesting increased IFN$\alpha$ was believed to be a local phenomenon. However, systemic activity of type I IFN was demonstrated using peripheral monocytes from pSS in which several genes associated with IFN exposure were demonstrated, and serum from patients had an enhanced capacity of inducing those genes in the monocytic cell line, suggesting type 1 IFN activity is not only a local but also a systemic phenomenon and pDC may be a possible source of type I IFN in pSS [45, 48]. Interferon regulatory factor 5 (IRF5) and signal transducer and activator of transcription 4 (STAT4) gene polymorphisms in the activation of type I IFN and stimulation of innate immunity in mice resulted in dryness, which preceded inflammation in salivary glands, have been reported [49]. In addition, EBV can lead to innate immunity before the development of autoimmune epithelitis in animal models [41]. If that is the case, there is a possibility that circulating type I IFN in Sjögren's syndrome may affect function of lacrimal and salivary glands

The role of proinflammatory cytokines including inflammatory cytokines in Sjögren's syndrome pathogenesis will be introduced. In general, cytokines play a central role in the regulation of immunity and are often found to be dysregulated in Sjögren's syndrome [50]. Roescher et al. [51] reviewed that in the salivary glands, saliva, and serum of these patients many proinflammatory cytokines such as IFNs, interleukin (IL)-12, IL-18, TNF$\alpha$, IL-1$\beta$, IL-6, and B cell activating factor are upregulated, whereas anti-inflammatory cytokines such as transforming growth factor (TGF) $\beta$1 are undetectable or are expressed at relatively low levels in Sjögren's syndrome, except for IL-10. Baturone et al. [52] reported that patients with pSS showed significantly increased concentrations of each of the five cytokines (IL-1$\beta$, IL-6, IL-10, TNF$\alpha$, and IFN$\gamma$) in serum, when compared with the healthy control group, indicating the existence of an immune activation state. Serum levels of one of these cytokines, IL-6, were correlated with poor quality of life in these individuals. Willeke et al. [53] reported that the number of TNF$\alpha$ and IL-1$\beta$, but not IL-6, secreting peripheral blood mononuclear cells (PBMCs) was significantly higher in patients with pSS than in controls. Patients with recurrent parotid swelling (RPS) had a significantly increased number of IL-1$\beta$-secreting PBMCs. Moreover, the number of IL-1$\beta$-secreting PBMCs correlated with the disease activity with the increased concentration of IgM rheumatoid factor (RF) and IgG RF. Other autoantibodies did not correlate with cytokine secreting PBMCs. The increased systemic secretion of IL-1$\beta$ and TNF-$\alpha$ in patients with pSS points to a pathogenic impact of these cytokines in this autoimmune disease. In particular, the correlation of IL-1$\beta$-secreting PBMCs with RPS and RF production indicates that IL-1$\beta$ is a crucial regulator in the development of local and systemic disease manifestations.

Human salivary gland cells can be induced to express HLA-DR mRNA along with other inflammatory cytokine gene expression such as IL-1$\beta$, TNF$\alpha$, and IL-6, following stimulation with IFN$\gamma$ [54]. Furthermore, IFN-$\gamma$ is able to upregulate B7.1, B7.2, and HLA-DR expression in salivary gland epithelial cell lines from Sjögren's syndrome patients [12, 55]. These suggest a possible involvement of IFN$\gamma$ in triggering the epithelial pathology of salivary gland at a preclinical, asymptomatic phase in NOD mice, and active participation of epithelial cells in the disease process occurs through the expression or upregulation of co-stimulatory molecules for the presentation of antigen to the T-cell or through the upregulation of apoptotic molecules such as FasL to induce apoptosis in the diseased glands.

Yamakawa et al. [56] reported that IL-1$\beta$, TNF$\alpha$, and IL-6 have been implicated in the destruction of parotid gland acinar cells (but not duct cells) in autoimmune sialoadenitis. Yao et al. [57] reported that the intraperitoneal injection of lipopolysaccharide (LPS) induced the expression of mRNAs of IL-1$\beta$, IL-6, and TNF$\alpha$ in the submandibular gland of C3H/HeN mice but not that of C3H/HeJ mice, a mutant strain for lacking of Toll-like receptor-4 (TLR-4(-/-) mutant). The mRNA levels of these cytokines in the submandibular glands of the wild-type mice increased as early as 3 hr after injection, peaked at 3-6 hr, and had decreased again by 24 hr. IL-1$\beta$ proteins were localized in the secretory granules of granular convoluted tubular (GCT) cells in the submandibular gland, and IL-1$\beta$ of the same size appeared in the saliva 6 hr after LPS injection in C3H/HeN but not in C3H/HeJ mice. Also, the amount of IL-1$\beta$ protein is upregulated in acinar cells prepared from lacrimal glands infiltrated with lymphocytes, suggesting that elevated levels of IL-1$\beta$, as they occur in Sjögren's syndrome exocrine glands, may impair the secretory function of lacrimal glands. Cytokines especially proinflammatory cytokines may be involved in dysfunction of salivary and lacrimal glands by directly interfering with the epithelial cells in the glands during the phase of noninflammation other than autoimmune reaction. Moreover, it has been reported that, cytokines in the circulation may affect the function of epithelial cells [58], which may be related with decreased tears and saliva before the development of dacryoadenitis and sialoadenitis. Taken together, production of cytokines may affect function of those organs during the noninflammatory phases in sSS, including even in pSS with lesions of exocrine organs in the immune phase.

## 4. Acquired Immunity

A progressive loss of exocrine gland function due to glandular damage is induced by a lymphoid cell infiltration into these target organs. The autoimmune character of the disease and diagnosis in patients with Sjögren's syndrome are made by focal lymphocytic sialoadenitis in minor salivary glands with a focus score >1, defined as a number of lymphocytic foci (which are adjacent to normal-appearing mucous acini and contain more than 50 lymphocytes per 4 $mm^2$ of glandular tissue) with positive test for Sjögren's syndrome autoantibodies (SS-A/Ro and SS-B/La) in the serum [59]. Histopathology usually exhibits lymphocytic infiltration, with the majority of lymphocytes being CD4+ T cells in the minor salivary gland lip biopsy from Sjögren's syndrome patients in accompanying B lymphocytes [60-62]. Infiltrated lymphocytes are composed of mainly autoreactive CD4+ T cells [12], CD8+ T cells, and dendritic cells, and macrophages are also present, and T cells preferentially express the T cell receptor (TCR) V$\beta$6 and TCR V$\beta$8 in these tissues in an animal model [63]. In human lymphocytes consisting of T and B cells in the salivary gland lesions has been reported [64, 65]. Various studies indicate that human minor salivary gland biopsy tissue and salivary glands from mouse models exhibited helper T (Th) 1 type cytokine profiles at the sites of target organs. For example, in labial salivary gland of human patients with Sjögren's syndrome IL-2 and IFN-$\gamma$ mRNAs were consistently detected, whereas IL-4 and IL-5 mRNAs were detected in some cases associated with strong B cell accumulation, suggesting Th1 cells are essential in the induction and/or maintenance of Sjögren's syndrome, while Th2 cells are involved in the progression of the disease process, especially in local B cell activation [66]. Moreover, it has been reported that CD4+ T cells in salivary glands expressed large amounts of IFN$\gamma$ mRNA, whereas those cells produced little IL-4 and IL-5 mRNAs in Sjögren's syndrome patients [67]. Also lymphocytes infiltrating in the labial salivary glands of patients with pSS or sSS are capable of producing both Th1 and Th2 cytokines, and the balance between them shifts in favor of Th1 responses in large salivary glands with high infiltration score [68]. An increase in several proinflammatory cytokines (mRNAs expression), including IL-1$\beta$, TNF$\alpha$, IL-6, IL-7, IL-10, IFN$\gamma$, and inducible nitric oxide synthase (iNOS) was demonstrated in the submandibular glands of NOD mice, which are originally reported as a model for insulin-dependent diabetes mellitus, a model for pSS with lymphocytic infiltrates [63]. Also, cytokine mRNA detected in lacrimal tissue was similar to that seen in the submandibular glands but appeared both earlier and more intensely [63]. Distinct subset of CD4+ memory effector T cells such as Th17 cells may play an important in various autoimmune diseases, including Sjögren's syndrome [69-72]. Moreover, IL-23/Th17 pathway has been implicated in Sjögren's syndrome pathogenesis in Ro52-null mice, which develops systemic autoimmune disease resembling human lupus [73].

Autoantibodies may also play a role in the pathogenesis. Serologically, the presence of rheumatoid factor, hypergammaglobulinemia, and antibodies to nuclear protein, such as SS-A/Ro and SS-B/La [44] as well as antibodies against $\alpha$-fodrin [75], carbonic anhydrase II [76], and MR3 [77] have been observed in the sera of Sjögren's syndrome patients. The later could play a pivotal role in secretory function in pSS [78]. In addition, there is a possibility that cryptic antigens recognized by T lymphocytes and antibodies in autoimmune pathogenesis including Sjögren's syndrome [79].

## Regenerating Gene (*Reg*)

The regenerating gene, *Reg*, was originally isolated as a growth factor from a cDNA library of rat regenerating pancreatic islets [80-82]. *Reg* gene expression has also been identified outside the pancreas. Subsequently, many *Reg*-related proteins have been identified in human and other animals. The *Reg* family genes constitute a multi-gene family consisting of four subtypes [83]. In human, 5 functional *Reg* genes, i.e., *REG I$\alpha$* [80, 81], *REG I$\beta$* [84], *REG III* [85], *HIP/PAP* [86, 87], and *REG IV* [88] have been isolated. Reg family proteins function as acute phase reactants, lectins, anti-apoptotic factors, and growth agents and include growth factors. These proteins are primarily involved in cell proliferation and differentiation, inflammation, diabetes, and carcinogenesis [83, 89]. Type I (and type II) Reg proteins are expressed in regenerating islets [83, 90, 91]. Type III Reg proteins have been suggested to be involved in cellular proliferation in intestinal cells, hepatic cells, and neuronal cells. Importantly, mouse Reg III was shown to be a Schwann cell mitogen that accompanies the regeneration of motor neurons [92], and Reg protein functions as a neurotrophic factor for motor neurons [93]. It was reported that REG I protein was expressed in ductal epithelial cells in the minor salivary glands (MSG) of patients with Sjögren's syndrome [94]. However, which *REG* family gene(s) were expressed in MSG in Sjögren's syndrome patients was obscured.

Autoantibodies against REG were found in some diabetic patients [95, 96]. However, the occurrence of autoantibody against REG in Sjögren's syndrome patients was obscured. Presence of autoantibody against REG might compromise regeneration of damaged ductal epithelial cells. Expression of REG could be a key event in autoimmunity. This hypothesis is supported by the fact that the autoantibody against REG retarded β-cell proliferation *in vitro* [95]. It was reported that the expression of *Reg* family genes was regulated by several factors such as nicotinamide [97, 98], glucocorticoids [97, 99], nutrient factors [100], IL-6 [91, 97], IL-8 [101], IL-11 [102], IL-22 [103], IFNγ [104], IFNβ [91], and CINC-2β [105].

In this section, we will introduce the over-expression of *REG Iα*, *IL-6*, *IL-8*, *IL-6 receptor*, and *gp130* mRNAs in MSG of Sjögren's syndrome patients and possible involvement of autoimmunity to REG in patients with Sjögren's syndrome.

## 1. REG / Cytokine / Chemokine in MSGs

We analyzed mRNA levels of all the *REG* family genes (*REG Iα*, *REG Iβ*, *REG III*, *HIP/PAP* and *REG IV*) in MSG of Sjögren's syndrome patients using quantitative real-time reverse transcriptase-polymerase chain reaction (qRT-PCR) (Figure 2) [106]. No *REG Iβ* mRNA was detected either in the control or the Sjögren's syndrome MSG. The mRNA levels of *REG III*, *HIP/PAP* and *REG IV* were not different between the control and Sjögren's syndrome MSG. In contrast, the mRNA level of *REG Iα* in the MSG of Sjögren's syndrome patients was significantly higher than that of control ($P$=0.036).

We then analyzed REG Iα protein expression in MSG of Sjögren's syndrome patients by immunohistochemistry. REG Iα protein was stained strongly in ductal epithelial cells in 28 of 53 samples (53%), whereas acinar cells were immunostained only in two samples for REG Iα (Figure 3a, b) [106]. In REG Iα-positive samples, the intensity of staining was not associated with the degree of inflammation, fibrosis or acinic atrophy. These results support the idea that *REG Iα* mRNA over-expression is associated with inflammation triggered by autoimmune disorders such as Sjögren's syndrome.

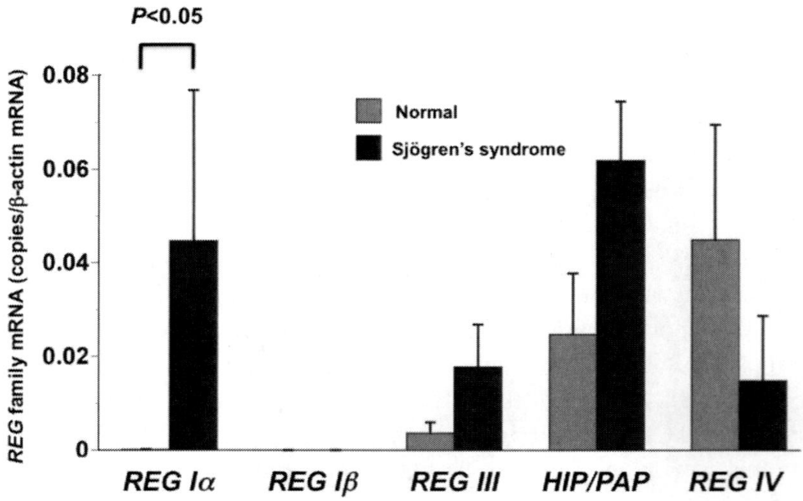


Figure 2. Expression of *REG* gene family in MSG (adopted from [106]). The mRNA level of *REG Iα* in the MSG of Sjögren's syndrome patients was significantly higher than that of control ($P$=0.036). *REG Iβ* mRNA was detected neither in the control nor the Sjögren's syndrome MSG. The mRNA levels of *REG III*, *HIP/PAP*, and *REG IV* were not different between the control and Sjögren's syndrome MSG. Data are expressed as mean ± standard error for each group (n=11-24).

It was reported that *Reg* gene expression was regulated by several factors, such as nicotinamide [97, 98], glucocorticoids [97, 99], nutrient factors [100], IL-6 [91, 97], IL-8 [101], IL-11 [102], IL-22 [103], IFNγ [104], IFNβ [91] and CINC-2β [105]. Among the major inflammatory mediators involved in the induction of inflammation of the salivary glands with primary Sjögren's syndrome, IL-6 is an important proinflammatory cytokine in relation to lymphocyte infiltration [107, 108]. In addition, the presence of IL-8 was reported in the salivary glands of Sjögren's syndrome [109, 110].

IL-6 and IL-8 are reported to induce *REG Iα* mRNA *in vitro* [97, 100, 101] and *in vivo* [111], and IL-11 [102], IL-22 [103], IFNγ [104], IFNβ [91] and CINC-2β [105] are also reported to induce *REG Iα* mRNA. IL-6R and gp130 are known as signal transducers of IL-6. We measured *IL-6*, *IL-8 IL-11*, *IL-22*, *IL-22R*, *IFNγ*, *IFNβ*, *CXCL1* (human homologue of *CINC-2β*), *IL-6R* and *gp130* mRNAs in the MSG by qRT-PCR [106]. As shown in Figure 4a, the *IL-6* mRNA level in the Sjögren's syndrome MSG was significantly higher than that in normal MSG. The *IL-8* mRNA level in Sjögren's syndrome MSG was also higher than that in normal MSG (Figure 4b). The mRNA levels of *IL-11*, *IL-22*, *IL-22R*, *IFNγ*, *CXCL1*, *IL-6R* and *gp130* in MSG were not significantly different between Sjögren's syndrome patients and normal control (Figure 4c-j). The mRNA of *IFNβ* was not detected in Sjögren's syndrome MSG (Figure 4g).

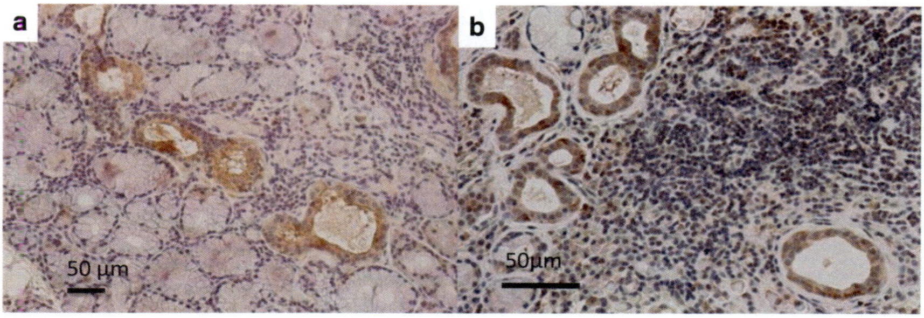


Figure 3. Immunostaining of REG Iα in MSG tissues (adopted from [106]). REG Iα expression was seen in regenerated ductal epithelia, together with a few inflammatory cells of heavily inflamed area from Sjögren's syndrome patients (a, b).

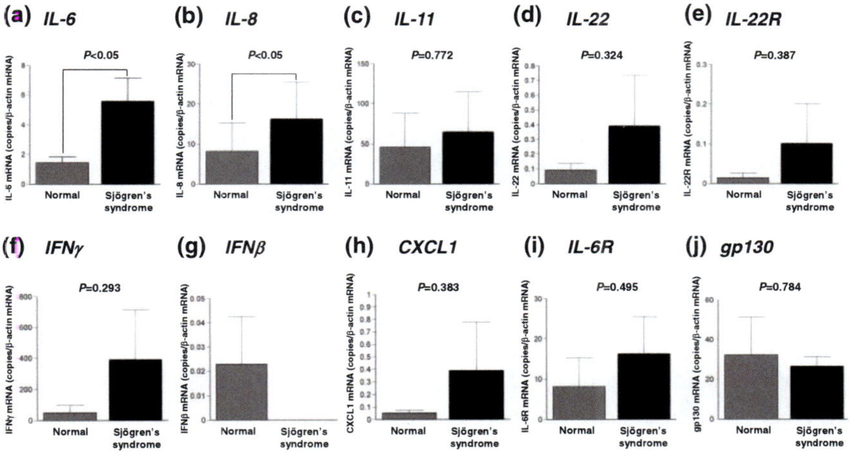


Figure 4. The mRNA levels of *IL-6* (a), *IL-8* (b), *IL-11* (c), *IL-22* (d), *IL-22R* (e), *IFNγ* (f), *IFNβ* (g), *CXCL1* (*CINC-2β*) (h), *IL-6R* (i), and *gp130* (j) in MSG (adopted from [106]). The mRNA level of *IL-6* in the MSG of Sjögren's syndrome patients was significantly higher than that of the control ($P$=0.0176). The mRNA level of *IL-8* in the MSG of Sjögren's syndrome patients was also higher than that of the control ($P$=0.0353). The mRNA levels of *IL-11, IL-22, IL-22R, IFNγ, CINC-2β, IL-6R* and *gp130* were not significantly different between the two groups. Data are expressed as mean ± standard error for each group (n=21-23). The mRNA of *IFNβ* was not detected in Sjögren's syndrome MSG.

We performed correlation analyses of expression of cytokine mRNAs and *REG Iα* mRNA and found that IL-6 mRNA expression was correlated significantly with *REG Iα* mRNA expression (*P*=0.0018). These results suggest that the up-regulation of cytokines, especially IL-6 and IL-8, induces over-expression of the *REG Iα* gene in Sjögren's syndrome MSG. IL-6R and gp130 are known as signal transducers of IL-6. We examined the mRNA levels of *IL-6R* and *gp130* in Sjögren's syndrome and normal MSG. The mRNA levels of *IL-6R* and *gp130* were not significantly different between the two groups (Figure 3i, j), suggesting that the increase of IL-6 in the salivary gland of Sjögren's syndrome patients (Figure 3a) can function as a switch for the IL-6/gp130 signaling system to induce *REG Iα* gene expression.

## 2. Anti-REG Iα Auto-Antibody

Auto-antibody was detected by Western blot as described [95, 106, 112, 113, 114] (Figure 5). Briefly, recombinant human REG Iα protein (20 μg) [95] was electrophoresed on a 12.5% sodium dodecyl sulphate (SDS)-polyacrylamide gel (9 × 7 × 0.1 cm) with a constant current at 20 mA/gel for 100 min and electrotransferred onto a polyvinylidene difluoride membrane using a semidry electroblotter, as described previously [95, 112]. After blocking with 5% non-fat dry milk, the membrane was incubated with patient or control serum, which had been diluted 1,024-fold with 5% non-fat dry milk, using a screener blotter [95, 112, 113]. The membrane was then rinsed with phosphate buffered saline containing 0.1% Tween 20 and incubated with goat antihuman IgG labelled with horseradish peroxidase at 1/1,600 dilution. The signals were visualized using an enhanced chemiluminescent detection system, as described previously [95, 112, 113]. The band intensities from positive blots were analyzed and the density was standardized using the value of an internal control sample treated as a relative value, as described previously [95, 112].

The sera from 117 patients with primary Sjögren's syndrome and 271 controls were screened for Anti-REG Iα antibody. A percentile graph of the relative anti-REG Iα antibody values is shown in Figure 6. The relative anti-REG Iα antibody values for all controls, with the exception of six individuals, were within the mean ± 3 SD value. Henceforth, we treated this mean ± 3 SD value (3.9) of the controls as the cut-off value for all related data analyses. Eleven per cent (13 of 117) of patients with primary Sjögren's syndrome subjects tested positive for anti-REG Iα antibody, whereas only 2.2% (six of 271) were positive in controls (Figure 6).

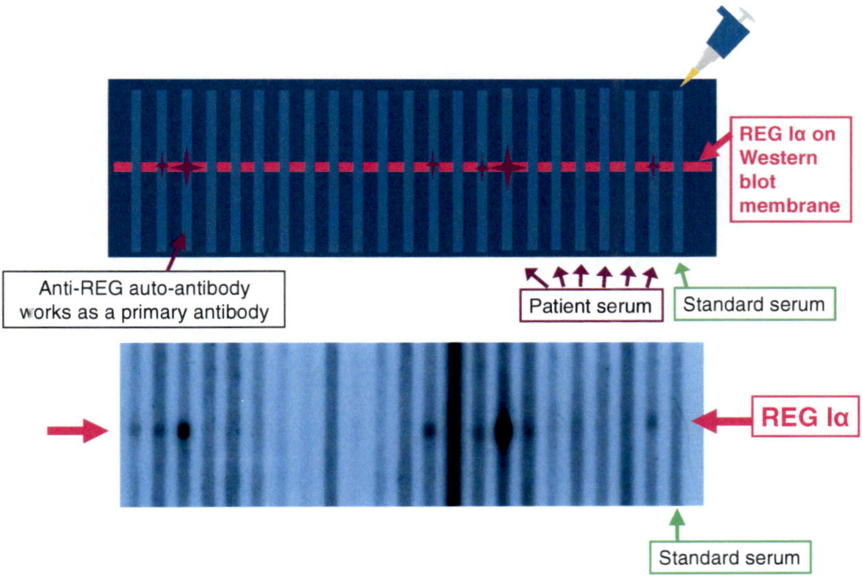


Figure 5. Schematic representation of anti-REG Iα auto-antibody measurement. Recombinat REG Iα protein [95, 97, 106, 115] was electrophoresed onto a 12.5% SDS-polyacrylamide gel with a constant current at 20 mA/gel for 100 min and electrotransferred to polyvinylidene difluoride membrane using a semidry electro-blotter. After blocking by 5% non-fat dry milk, the membrane was incubated with 1/1,024 diluted patient or control serum for 1 hr using screener blot (Screener Blotter Mini 56, Sanplatec, Osaka, Japan). The membrane was then rinsed with phosphate-buffered saline containing 0.10% Tween 20 and incubated with goat anti-human IgG labeled with horseradish peroxidase (American Qualex, San Clemente, CA) at 1/1,600 dilution. The signals were visualized by using an ECL detection system (GE Healthcare, Buckinghamshire, UK) as described [95, 106, 112]. The band intensities from positive blots were analyzed by Image J software (National Institute of Health, Bethesda, MD). The density was standardized using the value of an internal control sample treated as a relative value as described [95, 106, 112].

We evaluated the correlation between anti-REG Iα antibody and the clinicopathological factors of primary Sjögren's syndrome patients. The anti-REG Iα antibody-positive group showed significantly lower saliva secretion than the negative group using Saxon's test. The ratio of a destructive stage (stage 4 based on Rubin and Holt's criteria) in sialography in the anti-REG Iα antibody positive group was significantly higher than that in the anti-REG Iα antibody-negative group. In the patients with pSS, no correlation was found in age, sex ratio, serum levels of SS-A/SS-B autoantibody, anti-nuclear antibody titer, rheumatoid factor, amylase, IgG and HbA1c between the anti-REG Iα antibody-positive group and the anti-REG Iα antibody-negative group. Kerato-conjunctivitis sicca, Schirmer's test, also showed no significant difference between the two groups.

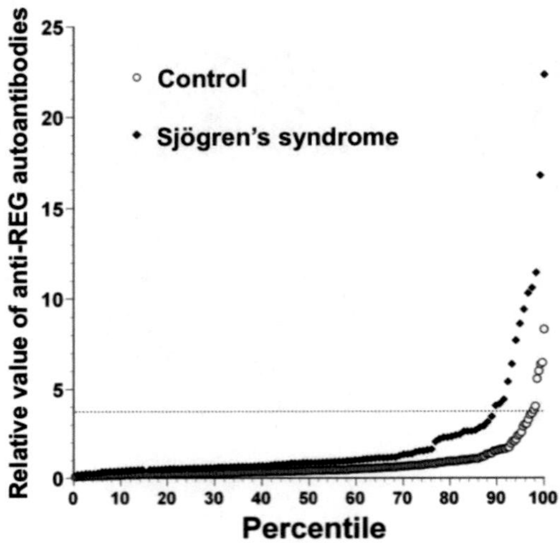


Figure 6. Distribution of anti-REG Iα auto-antibody in primary Sjögren's syndrome patients (adopted from [106]). The relative values from Western blot analyses of anti-REG Iα auto-antibody in 117 patients with primary Sjögren's syndrome patients and 271 control subjects are shown in percentile graph. Broken line indicates mean+3 SD (3.9) of the control samples and values above the mean+3 SD were regarded as autoantibody-positive.

In the histological features of labial salivary gland biopsy according to Greenspan's grade, there was no significant difference in the anti-REG Iα antibody-positive and the anti-REG Iα antibody-negative groups. We also examined extraglandular disease, systemic or severe disease (skin rash, Raynaud's phenomenon, arthralgia, thyroid gland disease, interstitial pneumonia, primary biliary cirrhosis, renal tubular acidosis, peripheral neuropathy and lymphoma); there was no significant difference in the two groups.

The anti-REG Iα antibody-positive group showed significantly lower salivary secretion and a higher ratio of the destructive stage in sialography. REG Iα protein was expressed in MSG ductal epithelial cells from nearly half of Sjögren's syndrome patients, and some in MSG acinar cells. Interestingly, all the patients in the anti-REG Iα antibody-positive group showed REG Iα expression in MSG ductal cells, whereas only 40% in the anti-REG Iα antibody-negative group showed REG Iα expression in MSG. These results suggest that autoimmunity to REG is associated with the regeneration of the ductal epithelial cells of MSG in pSS patients.

When salivary glands are damaged by inflammation, REG Iα protein may be induced in progenitor cells for MSG ductal/acinar cells such as ductal cells for recovering damaged cell mass by regeneration. Accumulating evidence concerning development of the salivary gland suggests the stem cell population of salivary glands is present in the intercalated duct [116, 117]. Additionally, the proliferation of pancreatic β cell was reported to be attenuated by the diabetic patient sera containing anti-REG Iα antibody *in vitro* [95]. It is quite possible that anti-REG Iα antibody attenuates not only growth-promoting affects of REG to fully differentiated acinar/ductal cells but also regeneration of the stem cell population of salivary glands. As a result, salivary functions including saliva secretion could become worse in Sjögren's syndrome patients with anti-REG Iα antibody (Figure 7).

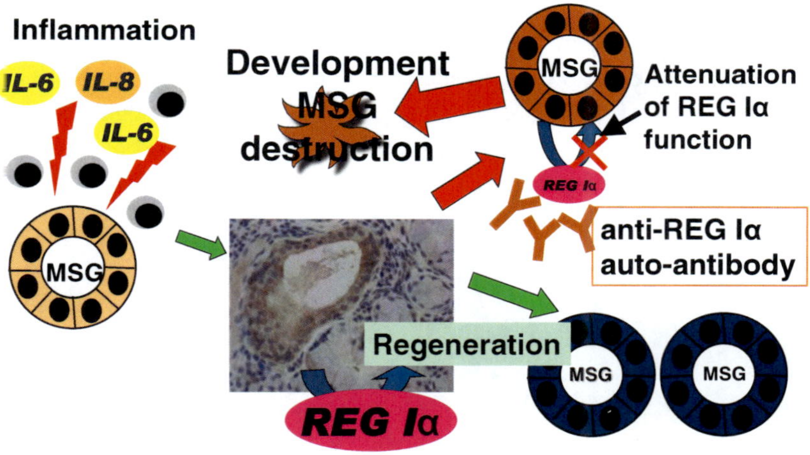


Figure 7. Possible role of anti-REG Iα auto-antibody in MSG destruction in Sjögren syndrome. The expression of REG Iα in MSG of Sjögren syndrome was significantly higher than that of the control, and the saliva secretion was significantly low in Sjögren syndrome patients with anti-REG Iα auto-antibody [106]. These results strongly suggest that autoimmunity to REG Iα is associated with the tissue injury of salivary glands in at least some Sjögren syndrome patients. When salivary glands are damaged by inflammation, REG Iα protein is induced in acinar progenitor cells such as ductal cells to recover damaged cell mass by regeneration. In the presence of anti-REG Iα auto-antibodies, ductal epithelial cell regeneration by REG Iα protein is attenuated, and REG Iα-producing ductal epithelial cell are destructed by the antibodies. As a result, salivary function goes worse in Sjögren syndrome patients with anti-REG Iα auto-antibodies.

Xerostomia is an important clinical concern in oral health and is known to induce various problems including dental caries, periodontitis, denture problems, mastication and swallowing problems, burning sensations, and dysgeusia [118]. Muscarinic agonist medications such as pilocarpine and cevimeline induced salivary secretion from the residual functional tissue [119]. However, these medications provided temporary relief of symptoms and had a limited effect on the recovery of damaged tissues. Accordingly, the development of a novel treatment to restore or regenerate damaged salivary gland tissues is eagerly awaited. It is unclear whether or not a specific signal is required for the regeneration of salivary gland. REG Iα may be a candidate growth factor for regeneration of the salivary gland cells as hepatocyte growth factor is a well-known protein that promotes the regeneration of liver and even protects tissue from damages [120, 121]. Therefore, it is expected that the regenerative growth of ductal epithelial cells serves as a practical therapeutic approach for Sjögren's syndrome.

In the aspects of Sjögren's syndrome diagnosis, detection of anti-REG Iα antibody is not so powerful. However, as the correlation between the salivary functions and existence of serum anti-REG Iα antibody, the anti-REG Iα antibody detection can be a useful diagnostic marker for the prognosis of the salivary functions such as saliva secretion. In addition, as described in materials and methods, it is required very small volumes of serum (less than 1 μl) to detect anti-REG Iα antibody.

## Conclusion

The pathogenesis of Sjögren's syndrome remains elusive. Environmental, genetic, and hormonal factors may be involved in its pathogenesis (especially as the role of trigger), and in the past, researchers have focused on the immune responses especially T cell-mediated and humoral immunities in the histopathological lesion during the inflammatory phase of Sjögren's syndrome [122]. The key question in this review is new aspects of mechanisms relating to dysfunction of salivary glands. Regarding nonimmune mechanisms, apoptosis/nonapoptosis and abnormal expression/distribution of AQPs may be, at least in part, induced genetically. Alternatively, it has been suggested that genetic defect in production of neurotransmitter may underlay in the pathogenesis of saliva insufficiency [123]. In addition, exogenous environmental factors (viruses and bacteria) may activate innate immunity, resulting in productions of type I IFN and compliments. Circulating proinflammatory cytokines may induce not only dysfunction but also morphological changes at the ultrastructural level of salivary glands. The cumulative effects of each factor/change may induce decreased function of salivary glands without inflammation.

We stressed the possible involvement of *Reg* in regeneration and destruction of salivary gland acinar and ductal cells in Sjögren's syndrome. *Reg* gene product (Reg protein) is important in the pathophysiology of various human inflammatory diseases such as diabetes, inflammatory bowel disease(s), and Sjögren's syndrome. We focused how the salivary gland dysfunction is initiated and maintained, and how it can be regenerated or progressed mediated by *Reg* gene and Reg protein. We have shown that *REG Iα* mRNA was expressed in the Sjögren's syndrome patient salivary glands and that REG Iα protein was expressed in the ductal epithelial cells of MSGs from patients with primary Sjögren's syndrome. Saxon's test revealed clearly that saliva secretion was reduced in primary Sjögren's syndrome patients with anti-REG Iα antibody. Furthermore, there was a correlation between the presence of anti-REG Iα antibody and REG Iα protein expression on ductal cells of MSG. We accentuated that autoimmunity to REG Iα could play an important role in the regeneration of MSG ductal epithelial cells in Sjögren's syndrome.

The causes of hypofunction in salivary glands are complex. The future challenge is to distinguish nonimmunologic mechanisms from immunologic mechanisms in target organs in this unique disease. Identification of gene(s) being responsible for nonimmune pathogenesis using gene targeting models is another way [124]. To create an integrated model that can account for salivary and lacrimal glands hypofunction is ideal [125].

## References

[1] Anaya, J. M. & Talal, N. Arthritis and Allied Conditions. In a Textbook of Rheumatology 13th edn (ed. Koopman, W. J.). Baltimore: Williams & Wilkins; 1997; pp.1561-1580.

[2] Alamanos, Y., Tsifetaki, N., Voulgari, P. V., Venetsanopoulou, A. I., Siozos, C. & Drosos, A. A. (2006) Epidemiology of primary Sjögren's syndrome in north-west Greece, 1982-2003. *Rheumatology* (Oxford), 45, 187-191.

[3] Trontzas, P. I. & Andrianakos, A. A. (2005) Sjögren's syndrome: a population based study of prevalence in Greece. The ESOrDIG study. *Ann. Rheum. Dis.*, 64, 1240-1241.

[4] Bowman, S. J., Ibrahim, G. H., Holmes, G., Hamburger, J. & Ainsworth, J. R. (2004) Estimating the prevalence among Caucasian women of primary Sjögren's syndrome in two general practices in Birmingham, UK. Scand. *J. Rheumatol.*, 33, 39-43.

[5] Delaleu, N., Jonsson, M. V., Appel, S. & Jonsson, R. (2008) New concepts in the pathogenesis of Sjögren's syndrome. *Rheum. Dis. Clin. North Am.,* 34, 833-845.

[6] Venables, P. J. Sjögren's syndrome. (2004) *Best Pract. Res. Clin. Rheumatol.* 18, 313-329.

[7] Ramos-Casals, M., Loustaud-Ratti, V., De Vita, S., Zeher, M., Bosch, J. A., Toussirot, E., Medina, F., Rosas, J., Anaya, J. M., Font, J.; SS-HCV Study Group. (2005) Sjögren syndrome associated with hepatitis C virus: a multicenter analysis of 137 cases. *Medicine* (Baltimore), 84, 81-89.

[8] Katsifis, G. E., Moutsopoulos, N. M. & Wahl, S. M. (2007) T lymphocytes in Sjögren's syndrome: contributors to and regulators of pathophysiology. *Clin. Rev. Allergy Immunol.*, 32, 252-264.

[9] Manoussakis, M. N., Boiu, S., Korkolopoulou, P., Kapsogeorgou, E. K., Kavantzas, N., Ziakas, P., Patsouris, E. & Moutsopoulos, H. M. (2007) Rates of infiltration by macrophages and dendritic cells and expression of interleukin-18 and interleukin-12 in the chronic inflammatory lesions of Sjögren's syndrome: correlation with certain features of immune hyperactivity and factors associated with high risk of lymphoma development. *Arthritis Rheum.*, 56, 3977-3988.

[10] Moutsopoulos, H. M. (1994) Sjögren's syndrome: autoimmune epithelitis. *Clin. Immunol. Immunopathol.*, 72, 162-165.

[11] Voulgarelis, M. & Tzioufas, A. G., (2010) Pathogenetic mechanisms in the initiation and perpetuation of Sjögren's syndrome. *Nat. Rev. Rheumatol.*, 6, 529-537.

[12] Cha, S., Peck, A. B., & Humphreys-Beher, M. G., (2002) Progress in understanding autoimmune exocrinopathy using the nonobese diabetic mouse: an update, *Crit. Rev. Oral Biol. Med.*, 13, 5-16,.

[13] Humphreys-Beher M. G., Yamachika, S., Yamamoto, H., Maeda, N., Nakagawa, Y., Peck, A. B. & Robinson, C. P. (1998) Salivary gland changes in the NOD mouse model for Sjögren's syndrome: is there a non-immune genetic trigger? *Eur. J. Morph.*, 36, 247-251.

[14] Kong, L., Robinson, C. P., Peck, A. B., Vela-Roch, N., Sakata, K. M., Dang, H., Talal, N. & Humphreys-Beher, M. G. (1998) Inappropriate apoptosis of salivary and lacrimal gland epithelium of immunodeficient NOD-scid mice. *Clin. Exp. Rheumatol.*, 16, 675-681.

[15] Qi, G., Hua, H., Gao, Y., Lin, Q. & Yu, G. Y. (2007) Sialoadenitis progression in nonobese diabetic mice and its correlation with expression of apoptosis-associated proteins in salivary glands and serum IgG levels. *Chin. Med. J.*, 120, 1426-1431.

[16] Ohlsson, M., Skarstein, K., Bolstad, A. I., Johannessen, A. C. & Jonsson, R. (2001) Fas-induced apoptosis is a rare event in Sjögren's syndrome. *Lab. Invest.*, 81, 95-105.

[17] Fox, R. I. & Maruyama, T. (1997) Pathogenesis and treatment of Sjögren's syndrome. *Curr. Opin. Rheumatol.*, 9, 393-399.

[18] Dawson, L. J., Field, E. A., Harmer, A. R. & Smith, P. M. (2001) Acetylcholine-evoked calcium mobilization and ion channel activation in human labial gland acinar cells from patients with primary Sjögren's syndrome. *Clin. Exp. Immunol.*, 124, 480-485.

[19] Pedersen, A. M., Dissing, S., Fahrenkrug, J., Hannibal, J., Reibel, J. & Nauntofte, B. (2000) Innervation pattern and $Ca^{2+}$ signalling in labial salivary glands of healthy individuals and patients with primary Sjögren's syndrome (pSS). *J. Oral Path. Med.*, 29, 97-109.

[20] Van Blokland, S. C., Van Helden-Meeuwsen, C. G., Wierenga-Wolf, A. F., Tielemans, D., Drexhage, H. A., Van De Merwe, J. P., Homo-Delarche, F. & Versnel, M. A. (2003) Apoptosis and apoptosis-related molecules in the submandibular gland of the nonobese diabetic mouse model for Sjögren's syndrome: limited role for apoptosis in the development of sialoadenitis. *Lab. Invest.*, 83, 3-11.

[21] Dawson, L. J., Fox, P. C. & Smith, P. M. (2006) Sjögren's syndrome-the non-apoptotic model of glandular hypofunction. *Rheumatology* (Oxford), 45, 792-798.

[22] King, L. S., Yasui, M. & Agre, P. (2000) Aquaporins in health and disease. *Mol. Med. Tody*, 6, 60-65.

[23] Xiao, L., Ng, T. B., Feng, Y. B., Yao, T., Wong, J. H., Yao, R. M., Li, L., Mo, F. Z., Xiao, Y., Shaw, P. C., Li, Z. M., Sze, S. C. & Zhang, K. Y. (2011) Dendrobium candidum extract increases the expression of aquaporin-5 in labial glands from patients with Sjögren's syndrome. *Phytomedicine*, 18, 194-198.

[24] Kobayashi, T., Fujimoto, T., Yane, K., & Hosoi, H. (2013) Abnormal distribution of aquaporin-5 and lymphoid infiltration in salivary glands of primary Sjögren's syndrome. *J. Nara Med. Assoc.*, 64, 65-72.

[25] Steinfeld, S., Cogan, E., King, L. S., Agre, P., Kiss, R. & Delporte, C. (2001) Abnormal distribution of aquaporin-5 water channel protein in salivary glands from Sjögren's syndrome patients. *Lab. Invest.*, 81, 143-148.

[26] Beroukas, D., Hiscock, J., Gannon, B. J., Jonsson, R., Gordon, T. P. & Waterman, S. A. (2002) Selective down-regulation of aquaporin-1 in salivary glands in primary Sjögren's syndrome. *Lab. Invest.*, 82, 1547-1552.

[27] Tsubota, K. Hirai, S., King, L. S. Agre, P. & Ishida, N. (2001) Defective cellular trafficking of lacrimal gland aquaporin-5 in Sjögren's syndrome. *Lancet,* 357, 688- 689.

[28] Delporte C. & Steinfeld, S. (2006) Distribution and roles of aquaporins in salivary glands. *Biochim. Biophys. Acta*, 1758, 1061-1070.

[29] Sasaki, Y., Tsubota, K., Kawedia, J. D., Menon, A. G. & Yasui, M. (2007) The difference of aquaporin 5 distribution in acinar and ductal cells in lacrimal and parotid glands. *Curr. Eye Res.*, 32, 923-929.

[30] Krane, C. M., Melvin, J. E., Nguyen, H. V., Richardson, L., Towne, J. E., Doetschman, T. & Menon, A. G. (2001) Salivary acinar cells from aquaporin 5-deficient mice have decreased membrane water permeability and altered cell volume regulation. *J. Biol. Chem.*, 276, 23413-23420.

[31] Soyfoo, M. S., De Vriese, C., Debaix, H., Martin-Martinez, M. D., Mathieu, C., Devuyst, O., Steinfld, S. D. & Deporte, C. (2007) Modified aquaporin 5 expression and distribution in submandibular glands from NOD mice displaying autoimmune exocrinopathy. *Arthritis Rheum.*, 56, 2566-2574.

[32] Nishimura, H., Yakeishi, A., Saga, T. & Yamaki, K. (2009) Effects of cevimeline on the immunolocalization of aquaporin-5 and the ultrastructure of salivary glands in Sjögren's syndrome model mice. *Kurume Med. J.,* 56, 39-47.

[33] Konttinen, Y. T., Tensing, E. K., Laine, M., Porola, P., Törnwall, J. & Hukkanen, M. (2005) Abnormal distribution of aquaporin-5 in salivary glands in the NOD mouse model for Sjögren's syndrome. *J. Rheum.*, 32, 1071-1075.

[34] Nikolov, N. P. & Illei, G. G. (2009) Pathogenesis of Sjögren's syndrome. *Curr. Opin. Rheum.*, 21, 465-470.

[35] Taniguchi, T. & Takaoka, A. (2001) A weak signal for strong responses: interferon-α/β revisited. Nature Rev. Mol. Cell Biol., 2, 378-386.

[36] Rönnblom, L. & Alm, G. V. (2001) An etiopathogenic role for the type I IFN system in SLE. *Trends Immunol.*, 22, 427-431.

[37] Anaya, J. M., Mantilla, R.D. & Correa, P. A. (2005) Immunogenetics of primary Sjögren's syndrome in Colombians. *Semin. Arthritis Rheum.*, 34, 735-743.

[38] Båve, U., Nordmark, G., Lövgren, T., Rönnelid, J., Cajander, S., Eloranta, M. L., Alm, G. V. & Rönnblom, L. (2005) Activation of the type I interferon system in primary Sjögren's syndrome: a possible etiopathogenic mechanism. *Arthritis Rheum.*, 52, 1185-1195.

[39] Oxholm, P., Daniels, T. E. & Bendtzen, K. (1992) Cytokine expression in labial salivary glands from patients with primary Sjögren's syndrome. *Autoimmunity*, 12, 185-191.

[40] Ittah, M., Miceli-Richard, C., Gottenberg, J. E., Sellam, J., Eid, P., Lebon, P., Pallier, C., Lepajolec, C. & Mariette, X. (2008) Viruses induce high expression of BAFF by salivary gland epithelial cells through TLR- and type-I IFN-dependent and -independent pathways. *Eur. J. Immunol.*, 38, 1058-1064.

[41] Horwitz, D. A., Zheng, S. G., Wang, J. & Gray, J. D. (2008) Critical role of IL-2 and TGF-β in generation, function and stabilization of $Foxp3^+$ $CD4^+$ Treg. *Eur. J. Immunol.*, 38, 912-915.

[42] Banchereau, J. & Pascual, V. (2006) Type I interferon in systemic lupus erythematosus and other autoimmune diseases. *Immunity*, 25, 383-392.

[43] Deshmukh, U. S., Nandula, S. R., Thimmalapura, P. R., Scindia, Y. M. & Bagavant, H. (2009) Activation of innate immune responses through Toll-like receptor 3 causes a rapid loss of salivary gland function. *J. Oral Pathol. Med.*, 38, 42-47.

[44] Gottenberg, J. E., Cagnard, N., Lucchesi, C., Letourneur, F., Mistou, S., Lazure, T., Jacques, S., Ba, N., Ittah, M., Lepajolec, C., Labetoulle, M., Ardizzone, M., Sibilia, J., Fournier, C., Chiocchia, G. & Mariette, X. (2006) Activation of IFN pathways and plasmacytoid dendritic cell recruitment in target organs of primary Sjögren's syndrome. *Proc. Natl. Acad. Sci. USA*, 103, 2770-2775.

[45] Wildenberg, M. E., van Helden-Meeuwsen, C. G., van de Merwe, J. P., Drexhage, H. A. & Versnel, M. A. (2008) Systemic increase in type I interferon activity in Sjögren's syndrome: a putative role for plasmacytoid dendritic cells. *Eur. J. Immunol.*, 38, 2024-2033.

[46] Moutsopoulos, N. M., Katsifis, G. E., Angelov, N., Leakan, R. A., Sankar, V., Pillemer, S. & Wahl, S. M. (2008) Lack of efficacy of etanercept in Sjögren's syndrome correlates with failed suppression of tumour necrosis factor α and systemic immune activation. *Ann. Rheum. Dis.*, 67, 1437-1443.

[47] Shiozawa, S., Shiozawa, K., Shimizu, S., Tanaka, Y., Morimoto, I., Yoshihara, R., Kuroki, Y., Hashimoto, M. & Fujita, T. (1990) Immunoreactive circulating alpha-interferon is low in Sjögren's syndrome. *Br. J. Rheumatol.*, 29, 50-52.

[48] Niewold, T. B., Rivera, T. L., Buyon, J. P. & Crow, M. K. (2008) Serum type I interferon activity is dependent on maternal diagnosis in anti-SSA/Ro-positive mothers of children with neonatal lupus. *Arthritis Rheum.*, 58, 541-546.

[49] Mariette, X. & Gottenberg, J. E. (2010) Pathogenesis of Sjögren's syndrome and therapeutic consequences. *Curr. Opin. Rheumatol.*, 22, 471-477.

[50] Szodoray, P., Alex, P. Brun, J. G., Centola, M. & Jonsson, R. (2004) Circulating cytokines in primary Sjögren's syndrome determined by a multiplex cytokine array system. *Scand. J. Immunol.*, 59, 592-599.

[51] Roescher, N., Tak, P. P. & Illei, G. G. (2009) Cytokines in Sjögren's syndrome. *Oral Dis.*, 15, 519-526.

[52] Baturone, R., Soto, M. J., Márquez, M., Macías, I., de Oca, M. M., Medina, F., Chozas, N., Garcia-Pérez, S. & Girón-González, J. A. (2009) Health-related quality of life in patients with primary Sjögren's syndrome: relationship with serum levels of proinflammatory cytokines. *Scand. J. Rheumatol.*, 38, 386-389.

[53] Willeke, P., Schotte, H., Schlüter, B., Erren, M., Becker, H., Dyong, A., Mickholz, E., Domschke, W. & Gaubitz, M. (2003) IL-1β and TNF α secreting cells are increased in the peripheral blood of patients with primary Sjögren's syndrome. *Ann. Rheum. Dis.*, 62, 359-362.

[54] Hamano, H., Haneji, N., Yanagi, K., Ishimaru, N. & Hayashi, Y. (1996) Expression of HLA-DR and cytokine genes on interferon-γ-stimulated human salivary gland cell line. *Pathobiology*, 64, 255-261.

[55] Manoussakis, M. N., Dimitriou, I. D., Kapsogeorgou, E. K., Xanthou, G., Paikos, S., Polihronis, M. & Moutsopoulos, H. M. (1999) Expression of B7 costimulatory molecules by salivary gland epithelial cells in patients with Sjögren's syndrome. *Arthritis Rheum.*, 42, 229-239.

[56] Yamakawa, M., Weinstein, R., Tsuji, T., McBride, J., Wong, D. T. & Login, G. R. (2000) Age-related alterations in IL-1β, TNF-α, and IL-6

concentrations in parotid acinar cells from BALB/c and non-obese diabetic mice. *J. Histochem. Cytochem.*, 48, 1033-1041.

[57] Yao, C., Li, X., Murdiastuti, K., Kosugi-Tanaka, C., Akamatsu, T., Kanamori, N. & Hosoi, K. (2005) Lipopolysaccharide induced elevation and secretion of interleukin-1β in the submandibular gland of male mice. *Immunology,* 116, 213-222.

[58] Zoukhri, D., Hodges, R. R., Byon, D. & Kublin, C. L. (2002) Role of proinflammatory cytokines in the impaired lacrimation associated with autoimmune xerophthalmia. *Invest. Ophthalmol. Vis. Sci.,* 43, 1429-1436.

[59] Vitali, C., Bombardieri, S., Jonsson, R., Moutsopoulos, H. M., Alexander, E. L., Carsons, S. E., Daniels, T. E., Fox, P. C., Fox, R. I., Kassan, S. S., Pillemer, S. R., Talal, N., Weisman, M. H. & the European Study Group on Classification Criteria for Sjögren's Syndrome. (2002) Classification criteria for Sjögren's syndrome: a revised version of the European criteria proposed by the American-European Consensus Group. *Ann. Rheum. Dis.,* 61, 554-558.

[60] Mavragani, C. P. & Moutsopoulos, H. M. (2010) The geoepidemiology of Sjögren's syndrome. *Autoimmun. Rev.*, 9, A305-A310.

[61] Mitsias, D. I., Kapsogeorgou, E. K. & Moutsopoulos, H. M. (2006) Sjögren's syndrome: why autoimmune epithelitis? *Oral Dis.,* 12, 523-532.

[62] Soyfoo, M. S., Steinfeld, S. & Delporte, C. (2007) Usefulness of mouse models to study the pathogenesis of Sjögren's syndrome. *Oral Dis.,* 13, 366-375.

[63] Robinson, C. P., Cornelius, J., Bounous, D. E., Yamamoto, H., Humphreys-Beher, M. G. & Peck, A. B. (1998) Characterization of the changing lymphocyte populations and cytokine expression in the exocrine tissues of autoimmune NOD mice. *Autoimmunity,* 27, 29-44.

[64] Humphreys-Beher, M. G. Brayer, J., Yamachika, S., Peck, A. B. & Jonsson, R. (1999) An alternative perspective to the immune response in autoimmune exocrinopathy: induction of functional quiescence rather than destructive autoaggression. *Scand. J. Immunol.*, 49, 7-10.

[65] Talal, N., Sylvester, R. A., Daniels, T. E., Greenspan, J.S. & Williams, R. C. Jr. (1974) T and B lymphocytes in peripheral blood and tissue lesions in Sjögren's syndrome. *J. Clin. Invest.*, 53, 180-189.

[66] Ohyama, Y., Nakamura, S., Matsuzaki, G., Shinohara, M., Hiroki, A., Fujimura, T., Yamada, A., Itoh, K. & Nomoto, K. (1996) Cytokine

messenger RNA expression in the labial salivary glands of patients with Sjögren's syndrome. *Arthritis Rheum.*, 39, 1376-1384.

[67] Fox, R. I., Kang, H. I., Ando, D., Abrams, J. & Pisa, E. (1994) Cytokine mRNA expression in salivary gland biopsies of Sjögren's syndrome. *J. Immunol.,* 152, 5532-5539.

[68] Mitsias, D. I., Tzioufas, A. G., Veiopoulou, C., Zintzaras, E., Tassios, I. K., Kogopoulou, O., Moutsopoulos, H. M. & Thyphronitis, G. (2002) The Th1/Th2 cytokine balance changes with the progress of the immunopathological lesion of Sjögren's syndrome. *Clin. Exp. Immunol.*, 128, 562-568.

[69] Katsifis, G. E., Rekka, S., Moutsopoulos, N. M., Pillemer, S. & Wahl, S. M. (2009) Systemic and local interleukin-17 and linked cytokines associated with Sjögren's syndrome immunopathogenesis. *Am. J. Pathol.,* 175, 1167-1177.

[70] Espinosa, A., Dardalhon,V., Brauner, S., Ambrosi, A., Higgs, R., Quintana, F. J., Sjöstrand, M., Eloranta, M. L., Ní Gabhann, J., Winqvist, O., Sundelin, B., Jefferies, C. A., Rozell, B., Kuchroo, V. K. & Wahren-Herienius, M. (2009) Loss of the lupus autoantigen Ro52/Trim21 induces tissue inflammation and systemic autoimmunity by disregulating the IL-23-Th17 pathway. *J. Exp. Med.*, 206, 1661-1671.

[71] Sakai, A., Sugawara, Y., Kuroishi, T., Sasano, T. & Sugawara, S. (2008) Identification of IL-18 and Th17 cells in salivary glands of patients with Sjögren's syndrome, and amplification of IL-17-mediated secretion of inflammatory cytokines from salivary gland cells by IL-18. *J. Immunol.,* 181, 2898-2906.

[72] Nguyen, C. Q., Hu, M. H., Li, Y., Stewart, C. & Peck, A. B. (2008) Salivary gland tissue expression of interleukin-23 and interleukin-17 in Sjögren's syndrome: findings in humans and mice. *Arthritis Rheum.*, 58, 734-743.

[73] Espinosa, A., Dardalhon, V., Brauner, S., Ambrosi, A., Higgs, R., Quintana, F. J., Sjöstrand, M., Eloranta, M. L., Ní Gabhann, J., Winqvist, O., Sundelin, B., Jefferies, C. A., Rozell, B., Kuchroo, V. K. & Wahren-Herlenius, M. (2009) Loss of the lupus autoantigen Ro52/Trim21 induces tissue inflammation and systemic autoimmunity by disregulating the IL-23-Th17 pathway. *J.* Exp. Med., 206, 1661-1671.

[74] Fox, R. I. & Kang, H. I. (1992) Pathogenesis of Sjögren's syndrome. *Rheum. Dis. Clin. North. Am.*, 18, 517-538.

[75] Haneji, N., Hamano, H., Yanagi, K. & Hayashi, Y. (1994) A new animal model for primary Sjögren's syndrome in NFS/sld mutant mice. *J. Immunol.*, 153, 2769-2777.

[76] Kino-Ohsaki, J., Nishimori, I., Morita, M., Okazaki, K., Yamamoto, Y., Onishi, S. & Hollingsworth, M. A. (1996) Serum antibodies to carbonic anhydrase I and II in patients with idiopathic chronic pancreatitis and Sjögren's syndrome. *Gastroenterology,* 110, 1579-1586.

[77] Bacman, S. R., Berra, A., Sterin-Borda, L. & Borda, E. S. (1998) Human primary Sjögren's syndrome autoantibodies as mediators of nitric oxide release coupled to lacrimal gland muscarinic acetylcholine receptors. *Curr. Eye Res.,* 17, 1135-1142.

[78] Bacman, S., Sterin-Borda, L., Camusso, J. J., Arana, R., Hubscher, O. & Borda, E. (1996) Circulating antibodies against rat parotid gland M3 muscarinic receptors in primary Sjögren's syndrome. *Clin. Exp. Immunol.,* 104, 454-459.

[79] Warnock, M. G. & Goodacre, J. A. (1997) Cryptic T-cell epitopes and their role in the pathogenesis of autoimmune diseases. *Br. J. Rheumatol.,* 36,1144-1150.

[80] Terazono, K, Yamamoto, H, Takasawa, S., Shiga, K., Yonemura, Y., Tochino, Y. & Okamoto, H. (1988) A novel gene activated in regenerating islets. *J. Biol. Chem.*, 263, 2111-2114.

[81] Watanabe, T., Yonekura, H., Terazono, K., Yamamoto, H. & Okamoto, H. (1990) Complete nucleotide sequence of human reg gene and its expression in normal and tumoral tissues. The reg protein, pancreatic stone protein, and pancreatic thread protein are one and the same product of the gene. *J. Biol. Chem.*, 265, 7432-7439.

[82] Watanabe, T., Yonemura, Y., Yonekura, H., Suzuki, Y., Miyashita, H., Sugiyama, K., Moriizumi, S., Unno, M., Tanaka, O., Kondo, H., Bone, A. J., Takasawa, S. & Okamoto, H. (1994) Pancreatic beta-cell replication and amelioration of surgical diabetes by Reg protein. *Proc. Natl. Acad. Sci. USA*., 91: 3589-3592.

[83] Okamoto, H. & Takasawa, S. (2002) Recent advances in the Okamoto model: the CD38-cyclic ADP-ribose signal system and the regenerating gene protein (Reg)-Reg receptor system in β-cells. *Diabetes*, 51, S462-S473.

[84] Moriizumi, S., Watanabe, T., Unno, M., Nakagawara, K., Suzuki, Y., Miyashita, H, Yonekura, H. & Okamoto, H. (1994) Isolation, structural determination and expression of a novel reg gene, human reg Iβ. *Biochim. Biophys. Acta, 1217*, 199-202.

[85] Nata, K., Liu, Y., Xu, L., Akiyama, T., Noguchi, N., Kawaguchi, S., Yamauchi, A., Takahashi, I., Shervani, N. J., Onogawa, T., Takasawa, S. & Okamoto, H. (2004) Molecular cloning, expression and chromosomal localization of a novel human REG family gene, REG III. *Gene,* 340, 161-170.

[86] Lasserre, C., Christa, L., Simon, M.T., Vernier, P. & Bréchot, C. (1992) A novel gene (HIP) activated in human primary liver cancer. *Cancer Res.*, 52, 5089-5095.

[87] Orelle, B., Keim, V., Masciotra, L., Dagorn, J.C. & Iovanna, J.L. (1992) Human pancreatitis-associated protein. Messenger RNA cloning and expression in pancreatic diseases. *J. Clin. Invest.*, 90, 2284-2291.

[88] Hartupee, J. C., Zhang, H., Bonaldo, M. F., Soares, M. B. & Dieckgraefe, B. K. (2001) Isolation and characterization of a cDNA encoding a novel member of the human regenerating protein family: Reg IV. *Biochim. Biophys. Acta,* 1518, 287-293.

[89] Zhang, Y. W., Ding, L. S. & Lai, M. D. (2003) Reg gene family and human diseases. *World J. Gastroenterol.*, 9, 2635-2641.

[90] Unno, M., Yonekura, H., Nakagawara, K, Watanabe, T., Miyashita, H., Moriizumi, S., Okamoto, H., Itoh, T. & Teraoka, H. (1993) Structure, chromosomal localization, and expression of mouse reg genes, reg I and reg II. A novel type of reg gene, reg II, exists in the mouse genome. *J. Biol. Chem.,* 268, 15974-15982.

[91] Planas, R., Alba, A., Carrillo, J., Puertas, M. C., Ampudia, R., Pastor, X., Okamoto, H., Takasawa, S., Gurr, W., Pujol-Borrell, R., Verdaguer, J. & Vives-Pi, M. (2006) Reg (regenerating) gene overexpression in islets from non-obese diabetic mice with accelerated diabetes: role of IFNβ. *Diabetologia*, 49, 2379-2387.

[92] Livesey, F. J., O'Brien, J. A., Li, M., Smith, A. G., Murphy, L. J. & Hunt, S. P. (1997) A Schwann cell mitogen accompanying regeneration of motor neurons. *Nature,* 390, 614-618.

[93] Nishimune, H., Vasseur, S., Wiese, S., Birling, M. C., Moltmann, B., Sendtner, M., Iovanna, J. L. & Henderson, C. E. (2000) Reg-2 is a motoneuron neurotrophic factor and a signalling intermediate in the CNTF survival pathway. *Nat. Cell Biol.*, 2, 906-914.

[94] Kimura, T., Fukui, H., Sekikawa, A., Yamagishi, H., Ichikawa, K., Tomita, S., Fujii, S., Imura, J., Kawamata, H., Chiba, T., Imai, Y. & Fujimori, T. (2009) Involvement of REG Iα protein in the regeneration of ductal epithelial cells in the minor salivary glands of patients with Sjögren's syndrome. *Clin. Exp. Immunol.*, 155, 16-20.

[95] Shervani, N. J., Takasawa, S., Uchigata, Y., Akiyama, T., Nakagawa, K., Noguchi, N., Takada, H., Takahashi, I., Yamauchi, A., Ikeda, T., Iwamoto, Y., Nata, K. & Okamoto, H. (2004) Autoantibodies to REG, a beta-cell regeneration factor, in diabetic patients. *Eur. J. Clin. Invest.,* 34, 752-758.

[96] Astorri, E., Guglielmi, C., Bombardieri, M., Alessandri, C., Buzzetti, R., Maggi, D., Velesini, G., Pitzalis, C. & Pozzilli, P. (2010) Circulating Reg1α proteins and autoantibodies to Reg1α proteins as biomarkers of β-cell regeneration and damage in type 1 diabetes. *Horm. Metab. Res.*, 42, 955-960.

[97] Akiyama, T., Takasawa, S., Nata, K., Kobayashi, S., Abe, M., Shervani, N. J., Ikeda, T., Nakagawa, K., Unno, M., Matsuno, S. & Okamoto, H. (2001) Activation of Reg gene, a gene for insulin-producing β-cell regeneration: Poly (ADP-ribose) polymerase binds Reg promoter and regulates the transcription by autopoly(ADP-ribosyl)ation. *Proc. Natl. Acad. Sci. USA.*, 98, 48-53.

[98] Kiji, T., Dohi, Y., Nishizaki, K., Takasawa, S., Okamoto, H., Nagasaka, S., Naito, H., Yonemasu, K. & Taniguchi, S. (2003) Enhancement of cell viability in cryopreserved rat vascular grafts by administration of regenerating gene (Reg) inducers. *J. Vasc. Res.,* 40, 132-139.

[99] Zenilman, M. E., Magnuson, T. H., Perfetti, R., Chen, J. & Shuldiner, A. R. (1997) Pancreatic reg gene expression is inhibited during cellular differentiation. *Ann. Surg.*, 225, 327-332.

[100] Qiu, L., List, E.O. & Kopchick, J. J. (2005) Differentially expressed proteins in the pancreas of diet induced diabetic mice. *Mol. Cell. Proteomics,* 4, 1311-1318.

[101] Yoshino, N., Ishihara, S., Rumi, M. A., Ortega-Cava, C. F., Yuki, T., Kazumori, H., Takasawa, S., Okamoto, H., Kadowaki, Y. & Kinoshita, Y. (2005) Interleukin-8 regulates expression of Reg protein in Helicobacter pylori-infected gastric mucosa. *Am. J. Gastroenterol.*, 100, 2157-2166.

[102] Lee, K. S., Kalantzis, A., Jackson, C. B., O'Connor, L., Murata-Kamiya, N., Hatakeyama, M., Judd, L. M., Giraud, A. S. & Menheniott, T. R. (2012) Helicobacter pylori CagA triggers expression of the bactericidal lectin REG3γ via gastric STAT3 activation. *PLoS One,* 7, e30786.

[103] Sekikawa, A., Fukui, H., Suzuki, K., Karibe, T., Fujii, S., Ichikawa, K., Tomita, S., Imura, J., Shiratori, K., Chiba, T. & Fujimori, T. (2010) Involvement of the IL-22/REG Iα axis in ulcerative colitis. *Lab. Invest.,* 90, 496-505.

[104] Sekikawa, A., Fukui, H., Fujii, S., Nanakin, A., Kanda, N., Uenoyama, Y., Sawabu, T., Hisatsune, H., Kusaka, T., Ueno, S., Nakase, H., Seno, H., Fujimori, T. & Chiba, T. (2005) Possible role of REG Iα protein in ulcerative colitis and colitic cancer. *Gut, 54*, 1437-1444.

[105] Kazumori, H., Ishihara, S., Hoshino, E., Kawashima, K., Moriyama, N., Suetsugu, H., Sato, H., Adachi, K., Fukuda, R., Watanabe, M., Takasawa, S., Okamoto, H., Fukui, H., Chiba, T. & Kinoshita, Y. (2000) Neutrophil chemoattractant 2β regulates expression of the Reg gene in injured gastric mucosa in rats. *Gastroenterology*, 119, 1610-1622.

[106] Yoshimoto, K., Fujimoto, T., Itaya-Hironaka, A., Miyaoka, T., Sakuramoto-Tsuchida, S., Yamauchi, A., Takeda, M., Kasai, T., Nakagawara, K., Nonomura, A. & Takasawa, S. (2013) Involvement of autoimmunity to REG, a regeneration factor, in patients with primary Sjögren's syndrome. *Clin. Exp. Immunol.*, 174, 1-9.

[107] Grisius, M. M., Bermudez, D. K., & Fox, P. C. (1997) Salivary and serum interleukin 6 in primary Sjögren's syndrome. *J. Rheumatol.*, 24, 1089-1091.

[108] Badillo-Almaraz, I., Avalos-Diaz, E., Villalobos-Hurtado, R., & Herrera-Esparza, R. (2003) FasL and Bax genes are differentially expressed in acinar epithelium and inflammatory cells of primary Sjögren salivary glands. *Minerva Med.*, 94, 341-345.

[109] Lee, Y. J., Scofield, R. H., Hyon, J. Y., Yun, P. Y., Lee, H. J., Lee, E. Y., Lee, E. B. & Song, Y. W. (2010) Salivary chemokine levels in patients with primary Sjögren's syndrome. *Rheumatology* (Oxford) 49, 1747-1752.

[110] Cuello, C., Palladinetti, P., Tedla, N., Di Girolamo, N., Lloyd, A. R., McCluskey, P. J. & Wakefield, D. (1998) Chemokine expression and leucocyte infiltration in Sjögren's syndrome. *Br. J. Rheumatol.*, 37, 779-783.

[111] Kiji, T., Dohi, Y., Takasawa, S., Okamoto, H., Nonomura, A. & Taniguchi, S. (2005) Activation of regenerating gene Reg in rat and human hearts in response to acute stress. *Am. J. Physiol. Heart Circ. Physiol.*, 289, H277-H284.

[112] Ikehata, F., Satoh, J., Nata, K., Tohgo, A., Nakazawa, T., Kato, I., Kobayashi, S., Akiyama, T., Takasawa, S., Toyota, T. & Okamoto, H. (1998) Autoantibodies against CD38 (ADP-ribosyl cyclase/cyclic ADP-ribose hydrolase) that impair glucose-induced insulin secretion in noninsulin-dependent diabetes patients. *J. Clin. Invest.*, 102, 395-401.

[113] Pupilli, C., Giannini, S., Marchetti, P., Lupi, R., Antonelli, A., Malavasi, F., Takasawa, S., Okamoto, H. & Ferrannini, E. (1999) Autoantibodies to CD38 (ADP-ribosyl cyclase/cyclic ADP-ribose hydrolase) in Caucasian patients with diabetes: effects on insulin release from human islets. *Diabetes,* 48, 2309-2315.

[114] Antonelli, A., Fallahi, P., Nesti, C., Pupilli, C., Marchetti, P., Takasawa, S., Okamoto, H. & Ferrannini, E. (2001) Anti-CD38 autoimmunity in patients with chronic autoimmune thyroiditis or Graves' disease. *Clin. Exp. Immunol.*, 126, 426-431.

[115] Kobayashi, S., Akiyama, T., Nata, K., Abe, M., Tajima, M., Shervani, N. J., Unno, M., Matsuno, S., Sasaki, H., Takasawa, S. & Okamoto, H. (2000) Identification of a receptor for Reg (Regenerating Gene) protein, a pancreatic β-cell regeneration factor. *J. Biol. Chem.*, 275, 10723-10726.

[116] Man, Y. G., Ball, W. D., Marchetti, L. & Hand, A. R. (2001) Contributions of intercalated duct cells to the normal parenchyma of submandibular glands of adult rats. *Anat. Rec.,* 263, 202-214.

[117] Man, Y. G., Ball, W. D., Culp, D. J., Hand, A. R. & Moreira, J. E. (1995) Persistence of a perinatal cellular phenotype in submandibular glands of adult rat. *J. Histochem. Cytochem.*, 43, 1203-1215.

[118] Atkinson, J. C., Grisius, M. & Massey, W. (2005) Salivary hypofunction and xerostomia: diagnosis and treatment. *Dent. Clin. North Am.*, 49, 309-326.

[119] Fox, P. C. (2004) Salivary enhancement therapies. *Caries Res.,* 38, 241-246.

[120] Ishiki, Y., Ohnishi, H., Muto, Y., Matsumoto, K. & Nakamura, T. (1992) Direct evidence that hepatocyte growth factor is a hepatotrophic factor for liver regeneration and has a potent antihepatitis effect in vivo. *Hepatology,* 16, 1227-1235.

[121] Nakamura, T., Nishizawa, T., Hagiya, M., Seki, T., Shimonishi, M., Sugimura, A., Tashiro, K. & Shimizu, S. (1989) Molecular cloning and expression of human hepatocyte growth factor. *Nature,* 342, 440-443.

[122] Kovács, L., Török, T., Bari, F., Kéri, Z., Kovács, A., Makula, E. & Pokorny, G. (2000) Impaired microvascular response to cholinergic stimuli in primary Sjögren's syndrome. *Ann. Rheum. Dis.*, 59, 48-53.

[123] Pedersen, A. M., Dissing, S., Fahrenkrug, J., Hannibal, J. Reibel, J. & Nauntofte, B. (2000) Innervation pattern and $Ca^{2+}$ signalling in labial salivary glands of healthy individuals and patients with primary Sjögren's syndrome (pSS). *J. Oral Pathol. Med.*, 29, 97-109.

[124] Manganelli, P. & Fietta, P. (2003) Apoptosis and Sjögren's syndrome. Semin. *Arthritis Rheum.*, 33, 49-65.

[125] Dawson, L. J. Fox, P. C. & Smith, P. M. (2006) Sjögren's syndrome-the non-apoptotic model of glandular hypofunction. *Rheumatology* (Oxford), 45, 792-798.

# Index

## A

## B



## C

## D

## E

## F



## G



## H

## I

## J



## K



## L

## M

## N



## O

## P

## Q



## R

## S

## T



## U